AMERICAN HEALTHCARE UNCHAINED

By Daniel Jones, MD

American Healthcare Unchained © **2012 by Daniel Jones, MD**

All rights reserved. No part of this book may be reproduced, stored in a retrieval system, or transmitted by any means – electronic, mechanical, photocopying, recording, or otherwise – without written permission from the publisher or author, except in the case of a reviewer, who may quote brief passages embodied in critical articles or in a review.

Dedication

~

This book is dedicated to my mother,
Nellie Jones, for her example of compassion,
service and courage.

And to my wife, Alicia, who gives me joy,
inspiration, and abundant feedback.

~

Table of Contents

~

Introduction 7

Chapter 1 – "Medi-Car" and the Demise of American Auto Repair 9

Chapter 2 - Healthcare Myths 23

Chapter 3 - Natural Laws Affecting Healthcare 43

Chapter 4 - How Healthcare Became Shackled — A Timeline 67

Chapter 5 - The PPACA (Obamacare) — Problems and Solutions 103

Chapter 6 - Unchaining American Healthcare 117

Conclusion 161

References 165

About the Author 171

Introduction

I graduated from medical school in 1980. Since then, I have practiced primary care medicine for 25 years, founded a successful online physician education company, and built a small-town primary care clinic.

When I applied for medical school in 1975, admission was fiercely competitive. Only 1 in 5 applicants was admitted. Medicine was regarded as the most prestigious profession a young person could enter — if you could get into medical school.

At that time, doctors enjoyed both high public esteem and the highest average income of all professions. Medicine was still regarded as the "noble profession." Little did I realize how the winds of change were blowing, and that my coveted profession would soon be in the eye of the storm.

To set the stage for an enlightened discussion of how American healthcare became as it is, and what we can do to improve it, I begin with a story. Chapter 1 describes what the car repair business would be like if mechanics were doctors.

Be forewarned: there are no heroes in this story. It is a tragedy. Like most tragedies, it is a story of good intentions with bad outcomes; of ordinary people facing extraordinary circumstances; of leaders not seeing the forest for the trees. Painful though it may be, let us examine the mistakes of the past, so that we may learn from them and chart a better path for the future.

I have good news as well. First, *there are no mysteries about how our healthcare system become what it is*. I will explain the reasons, motivations and historical events that have shaped today's healthcare system. Furthermore, *there are no mysteries about what is required to fix our healthcare system.*

Once you understand the causes of a problem, the solution becomes clear. *We can have abundant, convenient and affordable healthcare for all Americans.* This book explains how.

Chapter 1
"Medi-Car" and the Demise of American Auto Repair
An Allegory of American Healthcare

In the early 20th century, health care and automotive repair were similar service industries, supplied by thousands of small businesses all over America. In 1938, a teenager named Joe loved working on cars. When he finished high school, Joe got a loan and opened his own repair shop. He did good work for a fair price. Customers told their friends and neighbors. Soon Joe was getting busier, so he hired a receptionist and a junior mechanic. Life was good.

Then World War II began. Labor was scarce because most men were fighting overseas. Factories needed to attract workers, but couldn't offer higher pay due to the wartime wage freeze. Instead, they offered fringe benefits such as auto repair insurance.

Soon Joe was hearing from customers how they were being reimbursed by their insurance — even for routine things like brake jobs and oil changes. That seemed odd to Joe. Wasn't insurance for catastrophes, like a wreck or a blown transmission? Not anymore. Now it was being used as employee compensation. Consequently, it had to be something employees could "spend" on a regular basis.

At the time, car maintenance consumed less than 5% of GDP (Gross Domestic Product — the sum total of our nation's economic production), and nobody needed insurance just to maintain their car. Nonetheless, car repair insurance soon became a standard employee benefit, promoted by federal legislation in the form of tax incentives. That was soon to have unintended consequences, as we shall see.

One day, quite by accident, Joe's receptionist billed a customer's insurance $250 for a $25 brake job. Joe was surprised when, instead of an irate phone call from the customer, he got a check for $250 from the insurer — no questions asked. So he raised his prices. The insured customers didn't care as long as someone else was paying. Joe had discovered the insurance cookie jar. Thus was born the "consumer-payer disconnect," the seed of much mischief to come.

As the costs of repairs increased, employer-provided auto repair insurance became increasingly popular, allowing mechanics to raise prices further in a never-ending cycle. By the 1960s, it was becoming difficult for retired seniors on fixed incomes to keep their cars running. In response, Congress created Medi-Car, government funded auto repair insurance for seniors, financed by payroll withholding.

Seniors were often confused by the insurance claim forms, so Medi-Car decided to make mechanics bill Medi-Car directly. That further isolated customers from pricing and payment issues. The "consumer-payer disconnect" was now enshrined in law for Medi-Car, which soon became America's largest auto-repair insurer. All the mechanics signed up with Medi-Car, smiled, and dug deeper and more often into the cookie jar.

Before long mechanics were parking shiny new Cadillacs in front of mansions next to their bankers.

Joe and his fellow mechanics were happy. Medi-car customers were happy. But Congress was not happy. Medi-Car was becoming a real budget-buster.

Joe never expected the gravy train to last forever. He figured Medi-Car would eventually stop paying for non-catastrophic expenses and require customers to negotiate a fair price for major repairs before they were made, and then seek reimbursement. Those were the rules for most insurance plans. When that happened, he'd have to haggle about prices again and compete with Fred, the mechanic down the street. He might have to reduce his staff — maybe even downsize that mansion next to his banker — but he'd be OK.

That's not what happened. Congress seemed afraid to tell seniors they'd have to shop for an affordable mechanic, compare prices, and maybe even negotiate. Instead of restoring accountability and competition, Congress empowered Medi-Car to "control costs" by fixing prices and creating payment rules. Again, Joe was confused. He recalled the shortages, rationing, black marketeering and product adulteration that prevailed during the price controls of World War II. He recalled waiting half a day in a line of 200 cars to get gasoline during the Nixon price controls. What were the Medicare bureaucrats thinking? What were they smoking?

Now Medi-Car required Joe to provide a "CMT code" (Current Mechanic's Terminology code) for every item billed. With CMT codes, Medi-Car could tell exactly what they were paying for, and set prices and payment rules. Unbeknownst to Joe, Medi-Car bought their CMT codes from the American Mechanics

Association. Joe was still an AMA member then, and he trusted the AMA to look out for his interests.

By signing the Medi-Car contract, Joe lost control of his prices, but kept his senior customers. He grumbled, though, because after every job he had to search through a "CMT code catalog," bought from the AMA, to find the correct CMT codes for the bill. Otherwise, Medi-Car wouldn't pay.

If it weren't for the law of unintended consequences, this might have been where the story ends: Medi-car controls costs, and an acceptable status quo is reached. Alas, Medi-Car had overlooked an obvious pitfall: humans are smarter than monkeys, and even monkeys can find their cheese when you hide it under a coconut. Mechanics soon figured out how to manipulate the CMT codes to maintain their incomes.

Not to be out-smarted, Medi-Car upped the ante, making the rules more complicated. They added ADX codes (Auto Diagnosis Codes) to accompany the CMT codes. Only specific CMT codes were permitted with a given ADX code, and if they weren't matched perfectly, payment was withheld. When that didn't work, they added "modifiers" to make things even more tricky. Joe had to pore over 3-page decision flow charts to figure out which modifiers to combine with every CMT-ADX code combination. Without the correct modifier, payment was denied. Before Medi-Car, Joe's bills had been simple:

Front brake job. Labor: $60. Parts: $28. Total: $88.

With the new Medi-Car rules, that simple bill had to look like this:

Item Description	ADX Code	Mod-ifier	CMT Code	Price
Evaluation & Management – intermediate complexity	410.00	25	66213	$20.00
Replace front left brake pads:	410.01	50	61358	$12.50
Resurface front left brake drum:	411.12	51	61754	$5.50
Replace front right brake pads:	410.02	50	61358	$12.50
Resurface front right brake drum:	411.13	51	61754	$5.50
Left front brake pads (parts):	410.01	50	92173	$5.00
Right front brake pads (parts):	410.02	50	92174	$5.00
Brake fluid (supplies):	410.09	--	85261	$3.00
Flush front brake system:	410.09	--	23711	$7.00
Calibrate/adjust front brake system:	410.09	26	23915	$12.00
Total:				**$88.00**

If he didn't pair the *precise* ADX code from the thousands in his codebook (e.g., 410.01: "critically worn left front brake pads") and *just the right modifier*, with *every* CMT code on a bill, *exactly* according to Medi-Car's rules, Medi-Car refused to pay. Because the rules were complex and vague, Joe's bills were more often rejected than paid. He and his receptionist spent countless hours "correcting" and resubmitting bills.

Medi-Car's "Cost Control" Measures Drive Costs Relentlessly Higher

Since he had to spend so much time on billing, Joe wasn't able to fix as many cars. To compensate, he increased his fees again. That didn't help with Medi-Car because they only paid their fixed prices anyway. The private insurance companies paid his higher fees, but that wouldn't last long. And as prices got higher, his uninsured customers let their cars get in really bad shape before bringing them in. "Cost shifting" had begun.

Joe and his fellow mechanics now spent a *lot* more time on billing and collections. But once again, they found the cheese. For example, Medi-Car paid a basic "diagnostic fee" for each shop visit. So instead of doing a complete brake job in one visit, many mechanics would require customers to bring their car in *four times — once for each wheel!*

Mechanics soon developed an entire "toolbox" of similar techniques to maintain revenues at the cost of tremendous inefficiency and customer inconvenience. Now Medi-Car was paying not only for car repairs, but also for the "countermeasures" to combat their "cost control" measures. Joe's customers were paying with added inconvenience. And Joe was paying with strained customer relations.

With costs continuing to escalate, Medi-Car *really* needed to cut costs. So they came up with even more elaborate rules to reduce or deny payments. For example, if the brake pads had been replaced *anywhere* in the previous 180 days, they wouldn't pay. Of course, Joe had no way of knowing the customer's pads had been replaced at Fred's Garage 179 days earlier!

This situation spawned an entire new industry of "automotive billing and collections agencies." These businesses offered to handle all of Joe's billing and collections hassles for 10% of revenue. In spite of their claims, the agencies couldn't keep up with Medi-Car's sleight-of-hand either. All they did was collect the "easy bills," and then look for more mechanics to fleece, instead of figuring out how to collect the "hard bills."

It seemed that Medi-Car was finally winning its war with mechanics. After losing half his revenues for several years to one incompetent billing agency after another, Joe was going broke. But it was a Pyrrhic victory. Medi-Car's costs were still escalating due to the inefficiencies and counterproductive countermeasures they had spawned.

In desperation, Joe hired Toni, a "billing specialist." Toni had just graduated with a degree in "automotive coding" from one of the automotive coding schools that were popping up all over the country. Now, *finally*, Joe could get back to taking care of customers! But he couldn't help notice the irony: in addition to cutting the efficiency of his shop by half, Med-Car's "cost control" measures had now created an *entirely new business sector* (automotive billing & collection agencies), *and an entirely new profession* (automotive coding) for the auto repair industry to support! And more was yet to come.

Unfortunately, since Toni was a highly trained specialist, Joe had to pay her twice as much as his receptionist, Jill. Now he could barely pay himself. In desperation, he raised his fees yet again. That didn't affect what Medi-Car paid him, but at least he got more from the private insurance companies (more "cost shifting"). Business actually went down, though, because his uninsured customers just let their cars rust.

It wasn't long before the private insurance companies got wise: Medi-Car was paying less while they were being charged more due to cost shifting. A representative from BCBS (Blue Carb Blue Shocks, the biggest private insurance company) showed up one morning and demanded Joe sign a contract. He'd have to accept *their* fee schedule and payment rules if he wanted to continue serving their customers.

By now, Joe was nearing retirement age. Frustrated, he turned the business over to his son. Joe Junior wished he could tell BCBS to "shove it," but he was in a pickle. Many of his best customers had BCBS, the "Cadillac of car repair insurance." He couldn't afford to lose those customers, so he stuffed his pride and signed the contract.

Soon all the major insurance companies followed suit. That seemed unfair to Joe Jr. since the major insurers had millions of customers. That gave them tremendous bargaining power against "little guys" like Joe and his fellow mechanics. He felt powerless. Surely the American Mechanics Association would help.

But the AMA had other priorities. With mechanics hurting financially, fewer could afford the AMA's pricey membership dues. Meanwhile, the AMA needed to pay for its new high-rise headquarters and growing cabal of highly paid executives. Not to worry… the AMA had found the mother lode. On the one hand, they were making millions selling CMT codes to the government and insurance companies. Meanwhile, they were making millions more selling books, courses and software to desperate mechanics to help them cope with the ever-more-complicated codes and billing rules.

Like Medi-Car, once the private insurers had their CPT and ADX coding requirements in place, they too proceeded to "reduce costs" with complex rules to decrease or refuse payments. It wouldn't have been so bad if they all used the same rules, but *every insurer imposed a different set of rules*. It was impossible for Joe Jr. and Toni, his billing specialist, to keep up.

More "Cost Control" Measures Create Even More New Professions!

So Joe Jr. hired Anne, an "insurance verification and pre-authorization specialist" — yet another entirely new, highly trained and well-paid profession created by Medi-Car's "cost control" measures. Joe's personnel costs had now tripled. It was costing him more *just to get paid* than he was paying himself and his mechanics *to do the work!*

Even with all this help, Joe Jr. would often go unpaid for expensive jobs. The most egregious tactic was the requirement for "compliant documentation."

For example, one of Joe's customers had an accident, requiring a $4,000 repair. Instead of payment, though, Joe Jr. received a letter from BCBS stating, "After reviewing your records, we cannot find documentation that the rear bumper bolts had been tightened within the previous 3 years, per policy requirements. Therefore, the 40% of the car within 6 feet of the rear bumper is not covered. Furthermore, because the policyholder told the officer at the scene that he was 'just going to visit my mother on Mother's day,' the trip resulting in this accident does not appear to have been transportationally necessary. Therefore, this accident is not covered. If you wish to appeal this decision, please dial 1-800-WAITFOREVER and press option 4. You will then hear an announcement that you are 127th in line, and after 2 hours of 80's disco music, you will hear another message requesting you dial 1-800-WAITFOREVER and press option 4. Thank you for your business. We look forward to serving you in the future."

By now Joe Jr. was increasingly stressed, depressed, and disillusioned. He often wondered, was his life real — or was he living in the Twilight Zone? Nothing made sense any more. Why was he spending the majority of his time and energy playing cat-and-mouse games with faceless bureaucrats a thousand miles away, when all he wanted to do was fix cars?

Joe Jr.'s relationships with his staff and customers became strained. He was no longer able to diagnose and advise his customers over the telephone; with all the billing, coding, documentation and complex rules to follow, he was forced to spend every working minute on "billable activities" just to stay afloat. Meanwhile, his customers had no idea of the stress he was under. They assumed he was just greedy or grumpy. He sensed a loss of respect in the community.

Sadly, Joe Jr. realized his breed was dying out. To stay in business, mechanics were increasingly forced into large, "multi-specialty car clinics" in the larger towns and cities. That way they could obtain "economies of scale." Guys like Joe Jr. could no longer afford the army of insurance verification specialists, lawyers, accountants, billing specialists and coding specialists required to comply with the never-ending tsunami of laws, rules and regulations.

Although mechanics' incomes had been declining for decades, car care was now gobbling up 17% of GDP, nearly 4 times what is cost before WWII. It got so bad that some people had to sell their homes to pay for car repairs. If you were unfortunate enough to be uninsured, a transmission failure could result in bankruptcy. People were even shipping their cars overseas for repair. By 2010, you could take your car to Thailand, have a nice beach vacation *and* get your transmission rebuilt, all for half the cost of having it repaired in the US.

Something had to change. President Obama promised to fix auto care. Instead, he signed into law thousands more pages of rules and regulations and created another 159 bureaucracies to further "cost control," dictate, micromanage, complicate and constipate every aspect of the auto repair industry. To Joe Jr., it seemed Congress behaved like drunken sailors on a sinking ship, shooting more and bigger holes in the hull to "let the water out." Finally, at age 57, Joe Jr. admitted defeat and closed his shop.

Recall how this story began: "In 1938, a teenager named Joe loved working on cars. When he finished school, Joe got a loan and opened his own repair shop. He did good work for a fair price." That is still possible in America for mechanics, painters, plumbers, cosmetologists, accountants and lawyers. But for doctors and patients, those days are gone.

Chapter Summary

As illustrated in the preceding allegory, the major driver of healthcare inflation and inefficiency has been the *unintended effects and incentives* resulting from federal legislation and Medicare/Medicaid policies. I now capsulize that chain of unintended causes and effects in terms of patients and "providers" (doctors, clinics and hospitals):

- ➢ The wartime wage freeze and tax-favored status of insurance caused insurance to become a form of employee compensation, which **encouraged**...
- ➢ insurance to cover ordinary expenses, **resulting in**...
- ➢ the "consumer-payer disconnect" that **rewards**...
- ➢ doctors, hospitals and patients for using insurance as a "cookie jar," **causing**...
- ➢ rampant abuse of insurance and escalating prices, which **motivated**...
- ➢ Congress to create Medicare (initially another big cookie jar), that **exacerbated**...

- the consumer-payer disconnect and insurance abuse, thereby *motivating*...
- Medicare price-fixing and payment rules that *incentivized*...
- providers to focus on gaming the system instead of quality and affordability, *causing*...
- inefficient operations and further cost escalation, which *motivated*...
- Medicare to heap on even more "cost control" rules and regulations, which *spawned*...
- entire new industries and professions to cope with the added complexity, *causing*...
- costs of business for providers to skyrocket, *forcing providers to*...
- increase fees for private insurance and the uninsured (cost shifting), which *incentivized*...
- private insurers to demand contracted fixed fees similar to Medicare, which *resulted in*...
- uninsured patients, those least able to afford it, suffering the *greatest cost-shifting*!

That unhappy chain of unintended effects and perverse incentives continues today and will continue into the indefinite future, unless we make fundamental changes in our approach to healthcare financing. Note the major role of *unintended effects and incentives*. We will look at those issues in more detail later.

In this chapter, I emphasized the central role of Congress and Medicare in the decline of our healthcare system because I believe those are the most important factors. Several other factors have also been critical:

- The role of the AMA and other "special interest" professional and business organizations in restricting competition.
- The role of the FDA in restricting innovation and competition in drugs and medical devices.
- Our antiquated tort system that encourages litigation and defensive medicine.
- Laws that limit Americans' ability to sensibly control and prioritize their healthcare choices.

In the following chapters, we will explore these issues in more detail.

Chapter 2
Healthcare Myths

Before we can have an intelligent discussion about healthcare, it is imperative to dispel several "myths" that prevail in public discourse and the media. Like most enduring misconceptions, these myths are at least superficially plausible, and they support the agendas of specific interest groups or ideologies. On closer inspection, however, they turn out to be mere myths.

Myth 1: *"Technology drives up healthcare costs."*

As most people realize, in general, technology drives costs down, not up. For example, thanks to advances in technology, you can now get a personal computer 1,000 times more powerful than two decades ago for 1/10th of the cost. Similarly for home appliances, automobile accessories, cell phones, entertainment devices, etc. Technology normally drives costs down, not up — except when government becomes the primary payer, as in healthcare or military technology.

When I point out that technology normally drive costs down, proponents of this myth say, "Yeah, but healthcare is special." They point to the expensive new treatments and devices that didn't exist a few decades ago, such as hip joint replacements, implantable pacemakers, and automatic defibrillators. One doctor said, "The correct analogy is not that I have a bigger, better bicycle. Rather, I had a bicycle, but now I have a car." So let's look at new, as opposed to improved technology, in the non-medical world.

True, we did not have artificial hip joints and implanted pacemakers and defibrillators 60 years ago; but neither did we have most of the high-tech gadgets that now adorn our homes and cars — GPS systems, anti-lock disk brakes, air conditioning, microwave ovens, cell phones, wide-screen flat-panel TV's, etc. etc. Now we do, we take them for granted, and we pay for them as easily as we paid for much less 60 years ago.

When new gizmos are introduced, they're typically expensive, and only our wealthier or geekiest friends and neighbors have them. Within a decade or two, the price is down to a fraction (typically 10% or less) of the original price, and every teenager has one. How much have the prices on automatic defibrillators, MRIs and artificial joints come down? Not so much.

Why aren't we swimming in a similar cornucopia of increasingly numerous, wonderful *and affordable* medical devices? It's certainly not due to a lack of consumer demand, capital, or entrepreneurial spirit. No, *it's mainly due to the lack of a competitive free market in health care,* combined with the consumer-payer disconnect. (We touched on the consumer-payer disconnect in the allegory of Chapter 1 and will take a closer look later.)

In 1960, the typical middle-class family had one black corded phone and one car in the driveway (no garage), a gas stove, a fridge, a vacuum tube radio and a 12" B&W TV. Now you have a car for every driver, a cell phone for every talker, a double oven, side-by-side refrigerator-freezer, twin microwaves, food processor, espresso machine, kitchen-size barbecue grill on the deck, 55" flat panel LCD TV, tablet PCs, IPods, etc., *and you don't need insurance to pay for it.* Do you think that would be the case in the parallel universe where Congress took over consumer products instead of healthcare 50 years ago?

No, it is not technology, but government price-fixing, central bureaucratic management, and regulations preventing a competitive free market that are driving up healthcare costs. Consider the airlines and telecom industries. Before deregulation, we could only afford to call Grandma in Peoria on her birthday and holidays, and few people could afford to fly. Now, with competitive free markets, we call or email all over the world every day without even thinking about it. Similarly, when we plan a trip that takes longer than half a day to drive, we consider flying because it might be cheaper, overall. Isn't it time we considered unleashing the same creative forces in healthcare?

Myth 2: *"Fee-for-service is the problem; we've got to find a better way to pay doctors."*

A speaker recently commented, "We won't be able to stay within any sort of overall federal budget for healthcare, until we move away from our current fee-for-service payment system. This, more than anything, is the reason we can't control costs" [47].

Really? How is it possible not to notice that fee-for-service is, and always has been, a pillar of our formerly prosperous economy? Individual practitioners *setting their own fees and competing for customers* works just fine for cosmetologists, barbers, plumbers, appliance technicians and landscapers. It would probably work well in healthcare too — if we tried it.

Fee-for-service is the standard in virtually all professions and service industries: legal services, accounting, home appliance repair, plumbing, automotive repair — you name it. None of those industries has a problem with costs growing at twice the rate of inflation. No, the fundamental problem is not fee-for-service. The fundamental problem is that doctors and hospitals *are not free to set their own fees in competition for patients who are free to choose doctors and hospitals based on quality, reputation and price.* To force any kind of payment system on healthcare providers makes no more sense than forcing an arbitrary payment system on accountants, undertakers, plumbers or pet-sitters.

Elaborating on his warped reasoning, the above-mentioned speaker stated, "By basing payments on the volume of procedures — diagnostics, tests and so on…our fee-for-service system incentivizes providers and patients in all the wrong ways. The more procedures, the more revenue that goes to doctors and hospitals…" Does it not occur to those promoting this myth that *exactly the same dynamic* applies to any service industry you care to name? Why aren't those industries plagued with double-inflation, due to practitioners over-charging customers for unnecessary procedures and products?

The reason is simple: *in those industries the customer is the payer*, so the service providers must compete for his or her business based on reputation, quality and price. If a mechanic doesn't adequately explain the need for brake pads to be replaced, or replaces them unnecessarily, or over-charges, the customer tarnishes that mechanic's reputation and finds a new mechanic. In contrast, our current healthcare system prevents doctors from competing on price and quality, insulates patients from knowing or caring what is being paid, and forces patients to go to specific doctors who are "in network." It is those anti-competitive practices, *not fee-for-service*, that drive hyperinflation and inefficiency in healthcare.

When someone says, "The more procedures, the more revenue that goes to doctors and hospitals," the only logical response is "Obviously, and the decision as to what procedures I get and how much I pay should be between my doctor and me, not an anonymous bureaucrat who knows nothing of my condition."

As a final nail in the coffin of this myth, consider this: doctors rely on payment for services to pay their bills and put their kids through college, just like any other professional. Who is your doctor obligated to please in order to receive payment for those services? The answer is simple: your doctor is obligated to please whoever decides whether to pay him and how much. Would you prefer your doctor or hospital be obligated to please you, or your insurance company or Medicare?

Myth 3: "*Medicare is more efficient than private insurance.*"

This myth is based on the fact that Medicare doesn't spend nearly as much money as private insurance companies on marketing and recruiting patients, billing patients for premiums, collecting premiums, and financing business operations. Marketing, patient recruitment, premium billing, collections and financing (and the personnel to staff those functions) comprise the lion's share of non-medical expenses for any insurance company, including Medicare.

Unlike private insurance, however, the bulk of Medicare's administrative overhead is borne by other branches of the Federal government, and by America's employers and their accountants, through mandated employer withholding. Medicare's remaining administrative functions are mostly contracted out to private insurance companies such as BCBS and Cigna. It is therefore pointless to compare Medicare's overhead to that of private insurance companies. "Economists" who promote this myth are either deceitful (to promote an agenda) or incompetent.

Moreover, in my experience as a Medicare physician, I can attest that Medicare's rules regarding documentation, coding, pre-authorization, etc., *approximately double the net costs of providing care.* Those costs are not borne directly by Medicare, but are diffused throughout the system, borne by all players — hospitals, physicians and private insurance companies. Ultimately, of course, those costs are borne by patients and taxpayers.

According to Michael F. Cannon [22], "Economists who have tallied the full administrative burden of government health insurance programs conclude that administrative costs are far higher in government programs than in private insurance... Pacific Research Institute economist Ben Zycher writes that a 'realistic assumption' about the size of the deadweight burden puts 'the true cost of delivering Medicare benefits [at] about 52 percent of Medicare outlays, or between four and five times the net cost of private health insurance.' ...Medicare hides its higher administrative costs from enrollees and taxpayers, and public-plan supporters rely on the hidden nature of those costs when they argue in favor of a new government program."

For more discussion of these issues, please see "Is Medicare More Efficient Than Private Insurance?" by John Goodman and Thomas Saving at http://healthaffairs.org/blog/2011/08/09/is-medicare-more-efficient-than-private-insurance/

In summary, the assertion that Medicare is more efficient than private insurance is beyond mythical. It is a cruel hoax on American taxpayers, doctors and patients.

Myth 4: "*Solo and small medical practices are disappearing because big corporations are taking over America, and healthcare is just part of that process.*"

Big corporations have not taken over small business in America *except where they provide economies of scale that make small businesses uncompetitive.* You get a lot more options a lot quicker and cheaper at Walmart than you ever got at the Mom-and-Pop stores Walmart replaced. Do you get a lot more options a lot quicker and cheaper at the big multi-specialty clinics and hospital chains that have replaced the small clinics and community hospitals of yesteryear? Judge for yourself, but that hasn't been my experience. When I sold my medical practice to a multi-state hospital chain, the first thing they did was raise prices.

Big corporations have taken over healthcare because government over-regulation, price-fixing and central management have made it so inefficient that only large organizations can afford the army of lawyers, accountants, coders, billing specialists, and pre-authorization specialists now required to be in the healthcare business.

Our small towns and cities are still full of thriving solo and small-group legal, accounting, dental, and architectural firms, but that is becoming increasingly impossible for doctors. Are we wise to let our government continue the destruction of small practices, independent community hospitals, and entrepreneurship in healthcare?

Myth 5: *"Free markets don't work in healthcare."*

Advocates of "single-payer" or government-managed healthcare often promulgate this myth *but with no evidence to support it*. To prove this myth would require having a free market in healthcare that doesn't work. But we have not had a free market in health care since (arguably) the early 20th century, when healthcare was only 4.5% of GDP. Let's take a brief look at the history of healthcare.

Throughout the late 19th and early 20th centuries, the American Medical Association (AMA) grew in membership and influence. The AMA not only helped limit the supply of physicians, it also prevented competition among physicians by promulgating "usual and customary" fee schedules, and by prohibiting physician advertising or contracting. These flagrant anti-competitive practices continued until 1975, when the Supreme Court ruled in favor of the FTC's attempt to apply antitrust law to the professions.

That Supreme Court decision, which could have helped steer healthcare towards free-market competition, was made moot by the increasingly prominent role of private insurance and Medicare. By then, government-encouraged insurance abuse was already spiraling out of control, and Medicare was ten years old and embarking on its own program of price controls and central bureaucratic takeover of healthcare.

Numerous other federal and state laws and regulations implemented during the 20th century have constrained health care and insurance markets, as will be explained in more detail in a later chapter.

In summary: There has not been anything resembling a free market in healthcare in the modern era. The last time there *was* a semblance of a free market in healthcare, it consumed only 4.5% of GDP, not the approximately 18% that it consumes today. The assertion that "Free markets don't work in healthcare" is simply an unsubstantiated myth promulgated by special interests and ideology.

Myth 6: *"Electronic medical records will reduce costs."*

Electronic records *do* reduce costs and improve efficiency *in industries where they evolve naturally in response to industry needs* — such as banking, the airlines, and retail inventory. But in healthcare, because of bureaucratic regulations and price controls, electronic medical records have the opposite effect: they *increase costs and decrease efficiency*! Let me explain.

Instead of reimbursing whatever fee a doctor and patient have agreed on, Medicare (and most private insurance) dictates a fee-schedule that pays more for a complicated visit than for a simple visit. That seems reasonable, until you get to the next logical step and ask, "Well, how do you measure the complexity of a visit"? Unfortunately, the only way Medicare can assess the complexity of a visit is by the *complexity of the documentation* recorded for a visit or procedure. So to "game the system" for larger payments, doctors and clinics, hospitals, their billing agents, and the software companies who produce electronic records software, all dump ever-increasing amounts of worthless medical jargon into patient records. Doing so makes the services appear more complex, and thereby justifies larger payments.

If you could watch the sales presentation of any EMR (electronic medical record) vendor, you might be surprised by the sales pitch. Do they boast about how their EMR saves lives, reduces costs, and improves efficiency? Not much. No, mostly they boast about how their EMR allows you to create records that "support a higher level of reimbursement." Less euphemistically, their EMR creates "fat charts" for "fat payments."

With paper records, this chart-inflating practice is limited by the time and effort required to dictate or write lengthy records. *But it is amazingly quick and effortless for software to create reams of text.* In the old days, when a patient moved to a new doctor, their past medical records usually contained mostly useful information — assuming anyone could read it.

But nowadays, with electronic medical records, any meaningful information is usually buried in reams of worthless verbiage, whose sole purpose is to "beef up the chart" for better reimbursement. Increasingly, doctors don't bother to waste their time hunting useful information in these mostly worthless, inflated records. How can that good for healthcare? How can it possibly be good for the patient?

Even though electronic medical records have the *potential* to improve communication, efficiency, safety, and medical knowledge, in practice they often do the opposite because they are heavily "gamed" to justify higher charges. In fact, they often *decrease efficiency and safety* by making patient records practically worthless for their true purpose of communicating patient history and clinical information. This is a great example of two fundamental laws that are highly relevant to healthcare:

1. "People respond to incentives," a fundamental principle of economics.
2. The "law of unintended effects" that plagues all government attempts to micromanage our healthcare system.

We will explore these laws and their effect on healthcare in more detail in the next chapter.

In summary, electronic health records could and would improve quality and efficiency in healthcare, *if they evolved naturally, in response to business needs*, as in other industries. For that to happen, we must remove the perverse incentives that cause electronic health records to be designed and used primarily for ulterior purposes.

Myth 7: "*Healthcare is a right.*"

Myth 8: "*Healthcare is not a right.*"

During the Supreme Court hearings regarding the constitutionality of the Patient Protection and Affordable Care Act (PPACA, aka "ObamaCare"), Richard M. Salsman commented, "One need only read the legal briefs or hear the oral arguments made before the U.S. Supreme Court last week on the constitutionality of just one provision in the 2,700-page Obamacare law (the mandate to buy health insurance) to recognize that both sides blithely assume that 'health care is a right.' The law itself and many of the Justices also assume it. Thus most everyone in this alleged 'debate' is merely quibbling over how much the rights of health care providers will be violated – for that's what a mythical 'right to health care' entails" [14].

Salsman is most concerned about the rights of producers in society, and goes on to say, "…doctors, nurses, hospitals, researchers, drug-makers, or health insurers…are presumed to owe a 'noble' and selfless duty (i.e., their time, talent, income and profits) to patients; they are not at liberty to work on their own terms, but only on those dictated by demagogic politicians, or decreed by power-lusting regulators, or demanded by needy patients… Consumers allegedly have a 'right' to what health care providers provide, a 'right' to say what will be provided, when, and at what price…this is a form of slavery."

In contrast, it seems just as obvious to many on the left that healthcare *is or should be* a fundamental human right. Isn't it obvious that a caring society should take care of its less fortunate? When pressed regarding the negative effects of government largesse (e.g., violation of providers' rights, inefficient use of taxpayers' resources, and perverse incentives for the recipients), their response is often, "Oh, those right-wingers are so heartless."

Are those on the right of the political spectrum uncaring? Research seems to indicate otherwise. According to Arthur C. Brooks, a professor at Syracuse University, in "Who Really Cares: The Surprising Truth about Compassionate Conservatism," [26] liberals are markedly less charitable than conservatives:

- Though liberal families' incomes average 6 percent higher than those of conservative families, conservative-headed households give, on average, 30 percent more to charity.

- Conservatives give blood more often and donate more of their time.

- Residents of states that voted for John Kerry in 2004 gave less of their incomes to charity than did residents of states that voted for George Bush.

- People who reject the idea that "government has a responsibility to reduce income inequality" give an average of four times more than people who accept that proposition.

Of course, one could argue that liberals are just as charitable — only lazier. They want the government to do their charity work for them; and they don't mind paying more taxes to accomplish that. In my personal experience, it is more often the conservative physicians who staff free charity clinics, while liberal doctors rant online about how much we need a "single-payer system" (i.e., government-provided and controlled free healthcare for all).

The bottom line is this: both liberals and conservatives have compassion for the sick and poor. They just disagree about how to respond to their needs. Across the spectrum, there is consensus that the basic needs of all citizens should be met.

Therefore, the issue of whether healthcare is a "right" is moot. The real question is, "How can we ensure that healthcare is available to everyone who needs it *in the most efficient and affordable* manner possible, without violating the rights of others?" We are more likely to find consensus by approaching healthcare pragmatically, rather than by framing it as a political or philosophical issue.

Myth 9: "*Healthcare is special.*"

Myth 10: "*Healthcare is not special.*"

I've included this myth in both the positive and negative forms because it is actually true, but not in the way it is most often presented. The assertion that healthcare is special *because human health and lives are at stake* is often invoked as an emotional justification for extraordinary healthcare expenditures. In that sense, it is a myth, because housing, food, and many other factors besides healthcare per se are just as critical for human health and life. For example:

1. The most common cause of death and disability in Americans between the ages of 1 and 40 years is automobile accidents. The cost of the PPACA ("Obamacare") has been conservatively estimated to be at least about one trillion dollars over the next 10 years, and its net health benefit is questionable. Isn't it possible we could save more lives and prevent more disability if we spent that $1,000,000,000,000 dollars (or even 1/10th of it) improving highway safety?

2. Thirty percent of Americans are now officially obese, and obesity increases the risk of multiple serious and chronic diseases, including hypertension, diabetes, heart disease, stroke, degenerative arthritis and cancer. Meanwhile, starvation and under-nutrition are virtually non-existent in America. We could probably save a lot more lives, and prevent a lot more disability, if instead of spending $1,000,000,000,000 on the PPACA, we put a 50% tax on food and beverages.

   Given that Americans spend about 1.5 trillion dollars *every year* on food, if such a tax had the desired effect of decreasing total food consumption by 30%, it would not just improve Americans' health. Instead of *spending* $100,000,000,000 every year like the PPACA, it would actually generate over half a trillion dollars in annual revenue! (I'm not advocating a 50% tax on food, just pointing out how illogical our policy and spending priorities typically are.)

In truth, there is nothing special about "healthcare" per se, that justifies extraordinary expenditures relative to other initiatives to improve health and longevity, or to improve the quality of life.

In some ways though, healthcare *is special*, mainly with regard to how it is financed and insured. Consider a more typical type of insurance — say homeowner's insurance. Let's compare that with health insurance. (I'm talking here about *real* insurance: protection against catastrophic expenses.) How does homeowner's insurance differ from catastrophic health insurance?

1. **Spectrum of possible catastrophes:** With homeowner's insurance you need to protect against a relatively small number of catastrophic events: fire, tornados, lightning, hail, falling trees, and in some areas earthquakes, hurricanes and floods. With health insurance, on the other hand, you need to protect against a much larger spectrum of possible catastrophes, including numerous types of accidents, many diseases that might require expensive surgery, and many types of cancer, etc.

2. **Boundedness of total expense:** For homeowner's insurance, your maximum possible expense is the amount required to rebuild your home. With healthcare, the amount that could be spent on a catastrophic event is limited only by human creativity and willingness to spend.

3. **Variability of expenses with age and experience:** With homeowner's insurance, the fact that you've been hit by a tornado doesn't necessarily increase your future risk; and the risk of your house burning down doesn't necessarily increase as you get older. With health insurance, however, the older you are, the more likely you are to have major expenses; and a history of poor health indicates a higher risk of future health problems.

These factors complicate the issues of healthcare financing and insurance, but they are surmountable hurdles, as we shall see.

Myth 11: *"The more we spend on healthcare, the better our health will be."*

Much research shows this is simply not true [42]. Much of what we spend on healthcare has little if any marginal value, particularly when it is "free" to consumers. Take the much-touted "preventive care." As you must have noticed in the popular press, even the experts can't make up their minds whether or not it saves money or lives (not to mention all the time and worry) for women to get mammograms in their 40's, or for men to get PSA screening for prostate cancer.

Although we have spent enormous sums on Medicare, in truth it has not increased the longevity of our seniors [43]. Similarly, although people with high-deductible insurance spend 30% less on healthcare than those with first-dollar coverage, their health is just as good [44]. People with *no* insurance spend only about half as much, with no definite adverse impact on their health [38, 45]. Numerous lifestyle and environmental factors have been shown to have much greater effects on health and longevity than the amount of healthcare consumed — including diet, weight, physical activity, pollution, social status, smoking, and rural living.

Consider this: while the *marginal* gains in health disappear (or actually become negative) as we increase healthcare expenditures at the margin, the cost of that additional care *and the value of whatever else we could have purchased instead*, remains the same. For example, suppose you are a Medicare beneficiary, and you have arthritis in your hip. Suppose further that you and 20,000 other people, for whom Medicare would approve a hip replacement this year, aren't hurting all that badly. Maybe you would prefer to take a few extra Tylenol, and spend your hip replacement money on a new car, or a trip to Europe.

If Medicare or insurance is paying, it costs little or nothing at the time of surgery, so you will probably get that new hip. You can't get the new car or go to Europe instead, because you don't have the money — Medicare had to take it from you, one way or another, to pay for all those "free" hip replacements. You've been robbed of the choice of how to spend that money. Who would you rather decide how you spend your money, you or Medicare bureaucrats?

Myth 12: *"The PPACA (Obamacare) will reduce healthcare costs."*

There has been much debate over whether the PPACA will increase or decrease healthcare costs, based on estimates of the Congressional Budget Office

(CBO). The CBO's mandate is to provide congress with objective, non-partisan analysis of the budgetary implications of proposed legislation. Amazingly, the CBO's estimate *totally ignores* what is likely the greatest contributor to the PPACA's cost: *the enormous costs to doctors, clinics, hospitals, employers and insurance companies to implement and abide by the many thousands of new regulations emanating from the law and the 159 new bureaucracies it creates.* When you consider those costs, there is zero room for argument: the PPACA, like Medicare and Medicaid before it, will cause healthcare costs to rise far faster than general inflation. Congress has made *exactly this same budgetary mistake* consistently since the introduction of Medicare in the 1960s.

The cost of implementing and maintaining thousands of new regulations throughout an industry is enormous. The PPACA bodes well for the legal and accounting professions, and for all the new clerical and administrative positions that will be required to implement, enforce and monitor the new regulations. Even if the PPACA's new regulations increase the cost of healthcare only 5%, they will add another 1.1 trillion dollars in cost over the next 10 years, *at least doubling* the CBO's estimate.

Implementation costs aside, these regulations have not been carefully designed and tested by industry experts. Rather, they were hastily assembled by a Congress racing to meet an arbitrary political deadline. Furthermore, the PPACA does not constitute healthcare "reform" at all! It's just 2700 more pages of the same bureaucratic, heavy-handed micromanagement approach that Medicare and private insurance have been practicing for three decades — with spectacularly disastrous results. The only substantive difference is that now Congress has decided to bestow similar blessings on the insurance industry!

Conclusion: The Congressional Budget Office's estimate of the cost of healthcare reform only considered the government's *direct costs*. The Congressmen who passed this legislation, claiming it will reduce costs, *never considered the American healthcare industry's costs to implement this bill!* Those costs are enormous, and they will be passed on to the American public through higher costs, higher taxes, and diminished services.

Chapter Summary

In this chapter, I've attempted to dispel some of the myths surrounding the healthcare debate. However, it is equally important to understand some of the natural laws that have shaped our healthcare system. That is the subject of the next chapter.

Chapter 3
Natural Laws Affecting Healthcare

Before we consider what man-made laws might improve healthcare, it seems prudent to contemplate some relevant natural laws. Our man-made laws are unlikely work if they contradict the laws of nature. Worse, they might even backfire.

Natural Law 1: *"Changing a complex system has unintended effects."*

This is often called the "law of unintended effects" or the "law of unintended consequences." It is by no means confined to healthcare. We all create unintended effects every day. We do things to obtain some *intended* effect, but all too often, *unintended effects* cause us to regret our action.

Public policies and legislation often have adverse unintended effects [35]. Rent control is a classic example. In an attempt to increase affordable housing, some cities (e.g., New York) have enacted rent control legislation that prohibits landlords from raising rents. This usually results in (at least) two unintended effects:

1. When property owners are unable to raise rents to cover their rising costs, they are forced to neglect maintenance and improvements. If permitted to increase rents only when a new tenant leases, they've even been known to

intentionally make apartments unlivable for current tenants.

2. Real estate developers are unlikely to develop new housing where they have no ability to adjust rents to ensure a profit. This obviously results in less available housing, exactly the opposite of the intended effect.

In the Medi-Car allegory, we saw numerous unintended effects of government regulations, and analogous effects have occurred in healthcare. For example, when Medicare began requiring physicians to provide diagnosis and procedure codes, the intent was to limit unnecessary procedures, thereby reducing costs. But the unintended effect of increased complexity and business costs had the opposite effect.

The financial health of the medical industry became so dependent on proper coding that an entirely new profession was born, "certified medical coding," just to ensure that every medical bill was optimally coded. But wait… *there's more*!

With so much money at stake, America's growing army of college-trained "Certified Medical Coders" couldn't be trusted not to cook the books. Consequently, yet another entirely new profession — Certified Professional Medical Auditor (CPMA®) — has emerged, just to keep the coders honest!

To get an inkling of how much net expense Medicare's "cost saving" idea of medical coding adds to healthcare, just browse some of the 3940 search results for "medical coding" books on Amazon.com. A quick Google search for "degree in medical coding" illustrates the multitudinous ways you can become a well-paid member of one of these growing new healthcare "professions."

Today, whether or not you have Medicare, every time you pay a medical bill or a medical insurance premium, a significant fraction of that payment goes to support America's growing army of "certified" coders, billing specialists, insurance specialists and auditors. These positions contribute absolutely nothing to healthcare but cost, confusion, inconvenience and complexity. They exist for one reason: they are an *unintended consequence* of Medicare's most brilliant "cost saving" idea.

Not all unintended effects are bad; sometimes we are pleasantly surprised. In general, however, *the more complicated the system we alter, the more unintended effects we will create, and the more likely they will be harmful.* For example, suppose your bike isn't braking properly. A bicycle is a relatively simple system, and you can easily see that the brake caliper needs adjustment. If you're mechanically inclined, you might adjust the caliper yourself. Even if your adjustment causes some unintended effect — say an annoying squeaking sound — you can probably still ride your bike, and avoid the embarrassment of pushing it back home.

Now consider a more complex system. Suppose your computer isn't working properly. You might start by verifying that the cables are properly connected and the surge protector is on. If the problem persists you might consider opening the case and looking inside. The internal devices and circuitry are more complicated than your bicycle, and how it all works isn't so obvious. If nothing appears broken or misplaced, you might still be tempted to try a few things before taking it to the shop. Suppose you switch around a few of the wires connecting the various parts, close the case, and turn it on to test your "repair." What are the odds that your computer will work better than before?

Here's an important point about unintended effects: the likelihood of bad unintended effects outweighing the desired benefits is proportional to (a) the *complexity* of the system being changed, (b) our *ignorance* about that system, and (c) the *number or complexity of the changes* we make. Remember those three key aspects: complexity, ignorance, and amount of change.

Now consider something *really* complex, like our healthcare system. It's a system with literally millions of interconnected parts — clinics, doctors, hospitals, patients, insurance companies, pharmacies, etc. Clearly, our healthcare system has some serious problems and needs repair. Suppose a "committee" decides to fix it. Given the complexity of the system, the ignorance of the committee members, and the complexity of the changes they are introducing, what are the odds of bad unintended effects outweighing the intended benefits?

Does it help that our committee has a few economists and healthcare consultants? Not much, because economics isn't really a science in the same sense as physics or chemistry. No economist or committee of economists can "design" an economy (or an economic sector like healthcare), and predict its behavior the way an architect can design a skyscraper and predict it will not fall down. On a good day, the laws of economics can help explain what went wrong.

But you will study history a long time before you find an example of a "planned economy" that turned out as expected. (Please let me know if you find such an example.)

Let's recap. Our healthcare system is an extraordinarily large and complex system composed of many parts and players, each with their own agenda and interests. That's *high complexity*. We also have a relatively ignorant committee composed of lawyers, legislators, economists, and lobbyists, all under fiscal and political pressure to find a solution by an impossible deadline. That's *high ignorance*. Their solution (the Patient Protection and Affordable Care Act, aka Obamacare) is 2700 pages of changes, including the creation of over 100 *more committees* whose sole purpose is to monitor and create *even more changes*. That's *maximum change*. High complexity, high ignorance, and maximum change — we have all three. Now, what is the probability that the benefits of the PPACA will outweigh its adverse unintended consequences?

Natural Law 2: "*People respond to incentives.*" [35]

Why do people behave as they do? Some things we do out of habit. Sometimes we emulate childhood role models — good or bad. Sometimes we follow moral principles from our culture or religion. And many behaviors are just knee-jerk emotional reactions.

But most deliberate actions of rational adults are done *because we believe they will benefit us or those we care about*. We do what we expect will benefit us. For example, we get up when the alarm goes off, not because it feels good to drag ourselves out of bed. We do it because we know there are benefits for responsible behavior. As Adam Smith expressed it in 1776, "It is not from the benevolence of the butcher, the brewer, or the baker, that we expect our dinner, but from their regard to their own self-interest" [36].

Incentives are factors that cause people to believe a specific action will benefit them. The simplest examples are explicit rewards and punishments — things *intended* to change people's behavior. But many incentives are *not* intentional. We saw numerous examples in the Medi-Car allegory. Healthcare's problems are largely the unintended consequences of unintended incentives.

Case in point: when Medicare bureaucrats decided to compensate doctors based on the complexity of the documentation recorded, they created an incentive for doctors to create "fat charts." Consequently, the useful information in medical records is increasingly buried in reams of worthless verbiage. That's an *unintended consequence* resulting from an *unintentional incentive*. It is said that legal contracts are bloated with senseless lingo because medieval lawyers were paid by the page. Will we still be suffering the unintended consequences of the unintentional incentives of Medicare bureaucrats 500 years from now?

There are three important things to remember about incentives:

1. It is irrelevant what behavior the creator of an incentive intended to induce, or if they intended to create an incentive at all.

2. All that matters is that someone *perceives* an incentive, meaning that a particular behavior appears more or less likely to benefit them.
3. The effect of an incentive doesn't require any *conscious or cynical reasoning* by the person being influenced.

An honest doctor may not think, "I know I'll get paid twice as much if this chart is twice as long, so I'm going to beef this baby up big-time!" But it is naïve to think that honest people's behavior isn't influenced by ulterior motives inspired by perverse incentives.

Laws inevitably create unintended incentives, thereby causing unintended effects on behavior. Consider the law that makes employer-provided health insurance tax-deductible. That law provides a strong incentive for people to enroll in their employer's health plan. But because such plans are tied to a specific employer, and many employers *don't* provide insurance, an enrolled employee is strongly incentivized *not to change jobs*.

From an employer's point of view, that's a *good thing* — it improves employee retention. But the employee's fear of leaving a job because of health insurance considerations limits his or her mobility and employment opportunities. Ultimately, it limits employers' access to employees, and the ability of our labor supply to adapt to changing economic needs.

Natural Law 3: *"The Law of Supply and Demand"*

This law is fundamental to any discussion of economics, and is directly related to *economic efficiency*. Economic efficiency is a measure of people's ability to obtain the most of whatever they most want. The "law of supply and demand" describes how people naturally behave when competing to consume or provide goods and services.

One enduring theory asserts that maximum economic efficiency (the most goodies for the most people) results when the law of supply and demand is allowed to play out in a "free market" (where consumers are free to choose purchases based on their preferences, and suppliers are free to compete based on price, quality and reputation). That theory might or might not hold true, depending on environmental, cultural and regulatory variables. The law of supply and demand, however, is not just a theory. It is an inevitable consequence of the way we respond to incentives. It is a natural law that we ignore at our peril.

The law of supply and demand says that if you raise the price of an item (any product or service), then the demand (number of people willing to purchase) will decrease, because fewer people will be willing to pay the higher price. Conversely, if you lower the price, then demand will increase, because more people will be willing buyers at the lower price. It's that simple. When the price goes up, demand goes down; and when the price goes down, demand goes up.

Now consider the other side of the coin. Suppose there is a stable market for an item: manufacturers are producing just the amount to meet demand at the current price. How does a change in demand affect the price? For simplicity, we'll focus on "products," but exactly the same principles apply to services.

Suppose our product develops a great reputation, causing demand to increase: more people want it, and they want it more badly. With more people now willing to buy the product at its current price, stores will run out and inventory will be depleted. In a free market (where buyers and sellers are free to negotiate prices), usually two things will happen to bring supply and demand back into balance:

1. Stores will raise the price. At some higher price, fewer people will be willing buyers, and demand will go back down toward the amount being supplied.

2. Suppliers will notice they can now get a higher price. Therefore, they will be *incentivized* to invest in more machinery and personnel, to increase the supply.

Normally some combination of these outcomes will occur: the price will go up, but not so much as to decrease demand back to the original level; and production will increase to meet a higher demand. Thus, an increase in demand results in an increase in both price and supply (in the short run). Equilibrium, the product volume and price at which demand equals supply, is restored.

Conversely, suppose demand falls — perhaps a better substitute product comes on the market. When people buy less, the item accumulates on store shelves. In that case, stores and manufacturer will lower the price to get rid of the excess inventory. Since they can no longer get as good a price, suppliers will switch their production to other products with better profit margins. Some combination of lower prices and decreased production will again bring demand and supply into equilibrium. In more extreme cases the product becomes obsolete and is no longer produced.

When demand goes up, price and supply go up; and when demand goes down, price and supply go down.

By now you probably realize that our "law of supply and demand" actually involves *three* interdependent factors: supply, volume of demand, and price. Examples abound. Prices of heating oil rise in the winter and fall in summer. Drought causes the price of corn and soy to increase, thus increasing the cost of dairy and meat products. Lower labor costs overseas cause prices of manufactured goods to come down and demand to increase. These automatic adjustments are occurring constantly, resulting in an efficient market.

To summarize, if you start with a stable system, where demand equals supply at the current price:

1. When demand increases, prices go up (because sellers can charge more) and supply goes up (because producers can sell more and get a better price).

2. When demand decreases, prices go down (because sellers can't charge as much) and supply goes down (because producers can sell as much and get a worse price).

3. When price increases, demand goes down (fewer buyers are willing to pay the higher price) and supply goes down (because producers can't sell as much at the higher price).

4. When price decreases, demand goes up (more people will buy at the lower price). Supply may go up to meet demand, *if producers can still make a profit at the lower price*; otherwise, supply may go down as producers switch to more profitable products, *causing a shortage*, where demand exceeds supply.

5. When supply increases, prices tend to go down (sellers have to lower the price to sell more supply), causing demand to increase (more people are willing to pay the lower price).

6. When supply decreases, prices tend to go up (because buyers are competing for a smaller amount of goods), and demand tends to decrease (because fewer customers are willing to pay the higher price).

The law of supply and demand wasn't legislated by Congress, of course. It has been "discovered," in whole or in part, by multiple students of economics over many centuries, most famously by Adam Smith in his 1776 book, *The Wealth of Nations* [36].

The law of supply and demand is not a fundamental physical law like Einstein's $E = mc^2$. Rather, it results directly from the interaction of two basic human goals:

1. Buyers want to maximize the net benefit of their purchases, and

2. Suppliers want to maximize their profits.

It's not hard to see how the interaction of these two basic human goals results in the law of supply and demand as described — *if buyers are free to decide how to spend their money, and suppliers are free to adjust their prices and production.* In that situation, the law of supply and demand results in an *efficient market* (where supplier production is optimally matched to consumer needs and preferences), because freely fluctuating prices serve a critical communication function in the economy:

- The prices consumers are willing to pay for various items signal their needs and preferences to suppliers.

- The prices suppliers have to charge signal their costs of production to consumers.

When price signaling is prevented, as with Medicare price controls, the market becomes incapable of fluidly matching what suppliers produce to what consumers want. Economic efficiency is lost.

It is important to note that this law only describes how people *tend to behave when they have choices.* When their choices are restricted, the same tendencies are still there, but they may be expressed differently. For example, if demand for an item increases, but sellers are not allowed to raise the price, then suppliers will not be incentivized to invest in equipment and hire more employees to increase production. The store shelves will become empty, and frustrated would-be buyers will leave empty-handed.

Such situations are common in healthcare because Congress and the bureaucracies it creates routinely prevent the law of supply and demand from playing out naturally, to create economic efficiency. Our next law provides an example.

Natural Law 4: *"Price controls require rationing."*

It is vital to understand this simple law of economics, lest we be deceived by those who claim government bureaucracies can set prices for healthcare without rationing our care. We will soon see why this simple law can no more be circumvented than the law of gravity.

Those who advocate price controls in healthcare sometimes object to the free market out of fear that suppliers would set prices too high for some to afford care. That's a legitimate concern, but price fixing causes more problems than it solves. Here's how.

Suppose the price of item A (say, a drug or a medical procedure) is $100 and that's too high because some people who need it can't afford it. So let's assume the healthcare bureaucracy determines that the "fair" price for item A is only $50. What happens then? The law of supply and demand says clearly:

1. Because the price has gone down, demand will go up. More people will want to buy item A at the new price.

2. Because the profit margin on item A has decreased, suppliers will shift production to other products, and therefore produce less of item A than before.

Now, what happens when demand goes up at the same time that supply goes down? Suppose before the price went down, 100 people showed up at the store each week to buy the weekly supply of 100 units of item A. Now, 200 people show up to buy it at the new low price, but the manufacturer only sends 50 units because that's all he's willing to make at that price.

What do you call it when 50 items must be allocated to 200 willing buyers? It's called *rationing*. That's what happens when prices are fixed, as a direct result of the law of supply and demand. Anyone who says the government can set healthcare prices below free-market levels without causing rationing is either ignorant or lying. There is simply no other option.

It bears noting that Medicare and Medicaid have been price-fixing healthcare for several decades now, which has resulted in de-facto rationing via several mechanisms:

1. Many healthcare goods and services that patients want are simply "not covered." Because they are not covered, such products and services face monumental barriers to entering the marketplace. One consequence is that the US is losing its dominance in medical science and technology. Who will develop a new product or service when they know they cannot be paid for it because it's "not covered"?

2. Because *more* people want relatively *less* goods and services, medical resources *must be spread more thinly* across the pool of patients. The result is longer wait times for an appointment or procedure, longer wait times to see the doctor when you arrive for your appointment, less time

with the doctor, a smaller number of approved therapy sessions, a limited list of approved medications, tests, and treatments, etc.

Hence, medical goods and services are rationed by frank denial and by creating barriers to service, such as long waits, longer drives, and other inconveniences (repeated visits, pre-authorizations, appeals processes, etc.) [38].

At this point the astute reader, having mastered the Law of Supply and Demand, might see a solution for the rationing problem: in addition to controlling prices, why not also dictate production quotas? Unfortunately, even if our government decides to dictate how many doctors and nurses our schools must enroll, how many patients each doctor must see daily, and how many of each pill our pharmaceutical companies must produce, that still won't prevent shortages and rationing. That would require controlling *all three factors* involved in the law of supply and demand, *including demand — what you want and how badly you want it.*

We now understand how the government (via Medicare, Medicaid, or the new PPACA mandates) cannot control prices without causing rationing. You might say that rationing is preferable to letting suppliers set prices that are "too high." In fact, you might even point out that the free market also "rations" goods and services; it just rations them by price, rather than by outright denials and increased inconvenience or waiting.

Indeed, why not set prices and production quotas? Perhaps we can tolerate rationing if that would make everything "affordable." On the other hand, consider all the services you will necessarily be denied — that new non-surgical stem cell treatment for degenerative arthritis, or a new cancer treatment for a loved one. Think of the extra wait time, searching for an in-network doctor, forms to fill out, pre-approvals to request, denials to appeal, and so forth.

Would it be worth all that to make everything "affordable" and to ensure that prices are not "too high"? I have put "affordable" and "too high" in quotes, because it's important to examine those concepts more closely before we proceed. What does it mean for, say, a surgical procedure to be "affordable"?

Suppose you are uninsured (or have a very high deductible) and your shoulder has been hurting lately when you exercise. Your doctor says you need shoulder surgery that will cost $15,000. Is that "too high"? Maybe not, if you have an extra $15,000 of cash or available credit. Suppose, however, that your shoulder hurts mainly when you scrape the snow and ice off your windshield in the morning. Otherwise, it doesn't bother you much, so you'd rather forgo the surgery, and spend your $15,000 on a new garage instead. That way your shoulder won't hurt because you won't have to scrape ice and snow off your windshield, *and* you'll increase the value of your home by $15,000.

Would you rather decide how to spend that $15,000 yourself, or let some bureaucrat in Washington decide for you? Promoters of "government-paid healthcare for all" might say at this point, "Well, with Medicare-for-all, I could get the surgery for free, and keep my $15,000 to build a new garage." Unfortunately, Medicare-for-all can only pay for the surgery by extracting the $15,000 from you (or your friends, family and neighbors) through increased taxation or payroll withholding. You have to pay either way — what changes is who gets to decide how you spend your money.

At the end of the day, whether it is patients, employers, insurance companies or the "government" that pays, *our healthcare costs must be paid*. With the Medicare/PPACA approach, many choices are denied, and we have to pay for our healthcare not once, *but three times*:

1. We have to pay for the actual goods and services consumed.
2. We have to pay for the overhead and inefficiencies resulting from price-fixing and the perverse incentives of "control costs" measures.
3. We have to pay with our waiting times and inconvenience, because our time is money, and our wasted time reduces overall economic productivity.

There is even a fourth way in which we pay: by the deteriorating relationships with our doctors, nurses, and hospitals, who don't need to please us, the patients, but rather the payers.

The PPACA was sold to the public as a way of providing health services to the poor and uninsured. But how much care can we afford to give to the poor when our entire nation is *bankrupted by paying for everyone's healthcare at least three times*? Furthermore, there *will be a lot more poverty* because the exorbitant cost of healthcare is crippling our economy and our competitiveness in the global marketplace.

Because *price controls require rationing* (and cause numerous other perverse incentives and unintended effects), we see that a well-intended desire to create a fair and affordable healthcare system actually results in the opposite—the *most unfair and least affordable system of all*.

Natural Law 5: "*An efficient market requires low barriers to entry.*"

This simple law is best illustrated with an example. Suppose a new ointment has been created to treat baldness — balding people can rub it on their scalps to restore a full head of hair. Clearly, there would be a great demand for such a product.

Now suppose the ointment formula is posted on the Internet. All its ingredients are natural substances, not protected by patent, and are available for only a few dollars per pound. Furthermore, suppose there are no laws or regulations concerning who can make and market the product. What would happen?

Chances are that by sundown tomorrow, ten manufacturers would be hawking bottles of this new product for $99/ounce. Within a month, twenty companies would be making it, and the price would be down to $4.99/ounce. That's what happens with low barriers to entry: producers rush to fill an unmet need, at prices everyone can afford, because little time or investment is required.

Now consider what happens with high barriers to entry. Suppose the key ingredient is a complex molecule that only occurs in trace amounts in nature. The only way to create it in quantity is with a special "protein synthesizer" that costs $3,000,000. That's a technological and financial barrier to entry. Due to the high price of getting into the business, relatively few manufacturers would rush to produce the product, and they would have to charge a much higher price.

There are also regulatory barriers to entry. Suppose the FDA requires a special production license that costs $750,000 and requires filing out an application that won't be reviewed until the appropriate committee meets in nine months. Before the application can even be filed, the company is required to do a yearlong experiment with 1,000 patients to prove the product really works, and to investigate all possible side effects. Now, how many companies will produce this wonderful new product, how soon, and at what price?

Low barriers to entry encourage producers to deliver products and services more quickly, in larger volumes, at lower prices and in direct response to changing consumer demands. This equates to an efficient economy, where people's evolving needs or desires are readily met.

There are many types of barriers to entry. Some are natural and unavoidable, such as the cost of developing new products or training the providers of skilled services. Others are artificial, such as government regulations that increase the cost and delay of bringing new products to market or limit the supply of skilled service providers.

The law of supply and demand, operating in a free market, provides more efficient matching of productive capacity to consumer preferences than any other economic system discovered thus far. History shows just as clearly that a completely unfettered free market is inherently self-interested and shortsighted. Some degree of regulation is required to prevent abusive practices — monopolies, hazardous products, environmental degradation, etc. The trick is to find the optimal degree of wise regulation that allows the market to operate efficiently while minimizing abuses.

As we will see, too often government regulations are implemented in the heat of emotional reactions to specific abuses. Like most emotional reactions, they tend to be *overreactions*. The net result tends to be over-regulation, excessive barriers to entry, and an inefficient marketplace with unaffordable products, poorly adapted to consumer needs.

Natural Law 6: "*The quest for profits drives innovation and efficiency.*"

Why do people invest in mutual funds, stocks, bonds and real estate? Why do entrepreneurs build new factories and businesses, or improve current products and services? Why do inventors struggle to create new inventions?

It's a rare person who doesn't care about their community and environment. Most of us find comfort in the thought that our toils make the world a better place. Conversely, there is no faster, simpler recipe for depression than feeling useless. But when you look at economic behavior, the self-seeking motive appears to be the dominant force.

In discussions of healthcare reform it is common to see profits portrayed in a negative light. What repulses some people about profits seems to be these two attitudes or beliefs:

1. Profit seeking is a manifestation of *greed*, which we all know is *bad*. After all, it's one of the "seven deadly sins."

2. Taking profits out of the system makes the "profiteers" *wealthy* at the *expense* of everyone else.

"Greed" just refers to the excessive expression of our universal, innate human inclination to hoard resources today, so that we and our families are more likely to survive tomorrow. It is that desire to improve our economic situation that motivates both the buyer and the seller (i.e., the "profiteer") in any economic transaction. If the transaction is honest and mutually agreeable, then both parties benefit, and it is pointless to call either party "greedy." *The paying party receives a product he or she considers more valuable than the money paid; and the seller receives more money than his or her investment to deliver the product.* Any economic strategy that ignores or denigrates this basic human instinct to benefit ourselves in every economic transaction is doomed to fail.

Greed, in the pejorative sense of *excessive* self-interest that results in false advertising, product adulteration, or monopolization of markets, certainly is a bad thing. That is why we have laws to punish such activity. But it is critical to see the distinction between healthy self-interest and greed or *excessive* self-interest.

We wrestle with such distinctions every day in multitudinous ways. For example, the distinction between a healthy appetite that results in a healthy body, and the excessive appetite (pejoratively referred to as *gluttony*, another of the Seven Deadly Sins) that leads to morbid obesity. Or a healthy sexual appetite that leads to a healthy family, versus lust or lechery that leads to the Starr Commission.

We also have a universal human need, once our cupboard is stuffed, to reach out to our fellow man and share our wealth. That is why business titans like John Rockefeller, Dale Carnegie, the Walton family, Bill Gates, Warren Buffet, and many others go from wealth accumulation to wealth distribution and sharing. Both drives, as contradictory as they may seem, are part of our human nature. And both are beneficial to both individuals and our society, when properly channeled.

Another slur on profits sometimes encountered in discussions of healthcare reform is the notion of "excessive profits" or even "obscene profits." It's important to understand that "obscene profits" cannot be sustained in a free market. Here's why:

1. In a market where customers (or patients) are free to comparison-shop and purchase whatever appears to be the best product for the best price, someone charging enough to make an "obscene" or "excessive" profit simply won't be able to sell their product. People will find better bargains.

2. Suppose there are no "better bargains," just one supplier making "obscene profits." In that case, the profit-motive will cause other potential suppliers to enter the market as competitors,

charging something less, so they can attract customers and make a "slightly less obscene" profit. This process will continue until prices come down to a level that is consistent with prevailing returns on investment in other sectors.

It is also important to understand how profits (or actually, the *prospect* of profits) drive innovation and efficiency:

1. In a stable competitive market a supplier cannot make more profits by increasing prices, because that would only drive customers to buy from competitors.

2. Therefore, the only way to increase profits in a competitive market is to do one of the following:

   a) *Spend less* producing your product (i.e., *improve efficiency of production*), which ultimately allows you to charge less, and thereby attract customers from your competitors, or…

   b) *Improve the quality of your product* so that more people want to buy it.

Thus, a competitive market encourages suppliers to increase profits by either *increasing efficiency* or by *innovating to improve quality*. Over time, improvements in efficiency allow suppliers to make *the same profit by charging less*, and price competition forces them to do that, in order to attract buyers. In summary, *when suppliers are free to compete and buyers are free to shop*, the quest for profits leads to improved efficiency and quality, and to lower prices in the long term. *Everyone profits*, not just the "profiteers."

Chapter Summary

We have reviewed six natural laws of economics or human behavior that are highly relevant to healthcare:

1. *"Changing a complex system has unintended effects."*
2. *"People respond to incentives."*
3. *"The Law of Supply and Demand."*
4. *"Price controls require rationing."*
5. *"An efficient market requires low barriers to entry."*
6. *"The quest for profits drives innovation and efficiency."*

If you bear these laws in mind, it will be easier to understand succeeding chapters, where we discuss how healthcare came to be in its current state, and how we might most effectively improve it.

Chapter 4
How Healthcare Became Shackled — A Timeline

This chapter provides a timeline of key events that shaped our current healthcare system, with commentary on how those events relate to economic principles.

1890 and Before: The Wild, Wild West

Prior to the early 1900s, healthcare was so lightly regulated that "quacks" and "snake oil salesmen" ran amok in much of the country. In general, standards for medical education and licensure were light to nonexistent. Although "modern medical science" was beginning to offer some real benefits, most of the miracle cures we now take for granted, such as antibiotics, insulin, polio vaccinations, cardiac bypass and joint replacements, were yet to be invented. The public was widely abused by a multitude of uneducated charlatans, eager to take their money for worthless nostrums. Regulation was inadequate to prevent the rampant expression of "greed" in the marketplace. Honest and capable doctors existed, but patients had little ability to distinguish them from the more numerous quacks and pretenders.

1910: The Flexner Report

Widespread, unlicensed quackery was the state of affairs when the Flexner Report [27] was published in 1910, under the aegis of the Carnegie Foundation and the Council on Medical Education of the American Medical Association (AMA). That influential report emphasized that America had too many "physicians," most of whom were poorly trained.

The upshot of the Flexner Report was widespread reform and increased regulation:

1. Many medical schools closed, and educational standards for those that remained were greatly improved.
2. Physician licensure became much more strict and standardized, requiring more thorough training.
3. Medical quackery and charlatanism were greatly reduced.

Following the Flexner Report, the number of medical schools decreased by 80% and the per capita supply of physicians fell from 175 to 125 per 100,000 persons over the next few decades [32]. According to other sources, there were 131 medical schools in the U.S. in 1910, down to 76 in 1930, increasing to 85 by 1960, and then to 127 by 1981. Currently there are approximately 138 accredited U.S. and 17 accredited Canadian medical colleges. There are currently about 230 physicians per 100,000 persons in the US, which by no means represents a surplus.

Due to a combination of the Flexner Report and the AMA's consistent efforts to improve the organization and professionalism of American doctors, AMA membership and influence grew steadily throughout the early 1900s.

Currently all medical schools in the U.S. and Canada must be accredited by the Liaison Committee on Medical Education (LCME), a joint committee of the Association of American Medical Colleges (AAMC), the American Medical Association, and the Committee on Accreditation of Canadian Medical Schools (CACMS). All 50 states in the U.S. require M.D. candidates for medical licensure to be graduates of an LCMI-accredited medical school.

The Flexner Report and subsequent efforts by the AMA and other physician-led organizations resulted in substantial improvements in the quality of education and professionalism of American physicians. These improvements came at a high price, however: the supply of U.S. physicians was so tightly constrained that *from 1900 to 1975 the average incomes of physicians increased several fold relative to most other professions*. This is a clear example of the law of supply and demand: when supply is constrained, relative to demand, the price goes up.

Given the heavy involvement of the AMA and other physician-led organizations in the various reports and policy recommendations affecting physician supply, it is less clear whether the Flexner Report's effect on physician incomes is an example of the "law of unintended effects," or an example of leaders responding to incentives. In any event, since physician incomes account for only about 6% of healthcare costs, other factors are more important determinants of our total healthcare costs.

1914: The Harrison Narcotics Act

"In the 1890s the Sears & Roebuck catalogue, which was distributed to millions of Americans homes, offered a syringe and a small amount of cocaine for $1.50." [28] The same article further states, "At the beginning of the 20th century, cocaine began to be linked to crime. In 1900, the Journal of the American Medical Association published an editorial stating, "Negroes in the South are reported as being addicted to a new form of vice – that of 'cocaine sniffing' or the 'coke habit.'" Some newspapers later claimed cocaine use caused blacks to rape white women and was improving their pistol marksmanship."

The social circumstances that led to the Harrison Narcotics Act, and all the adverse unintended consequences that followed, are interesting because they represent the beginning of the erosion of Americans' right to control or manage our own healthcare. Prior to that act, if you had an abscessed tooth, a migraine headache or a broken toe, you could go to the corner pharmacy and get whatever you needed to control your pain until you could see your doctor, or otherwise manage your ailment as you saw fit. After this act became law, opiates (e.g., heroin, morphine, codeine) and cocaine were tightly controlled and could only be obtained by seeing a doctor or becoming a criminal.

While not advocating self-treatment, it's important to note that the right we once had to do so has been lost. The Harrison Narcotics Act also marks the ascent of "elitism" in American healthcare. The common person, regardless of education, could no longer care for herself, but instead was forced to rely on those with special certification. This trend has continued with subsequent laws, a few of which will be mentioned later in this chapter. Self-treatment is, of course, the most convenient and least expensive type of treatment. Laws that prevent it represent a high "barrier to entry" for millions of Americans who might otherwise give their doctors a little more competition.

Early 1900's: The Ascent of the AMA

The American Medical Association was largely responsible for improving the education, quality and professionalism of physicians in the late 1800s and early 1900s. As part of its efforts to improve professionalism and restrain charlatanism, the AMA promulgated a physician "code of ethics" that prohibited physician advertising, solicitation and contract practice. These prohibitions made sense in the context of the times. For example, charlatans and quacks often lured patients away from honest doctors by advertising miracle cures and discount prices.

Less clearly beneficial to the public was the AMA's publication of "usual and customary" physician fees, which restrained competition among physicians and facilitated the gradual relative increase in physician incomes. In 1975, my college economics professor railed against the AMA's anti-competitive practices. He claimed that, whereas doctors and college professors had equal incomes in 1900, by 1975 doctors' average incomes were *five times greater than his*.

The AMA's practice of restraining physician competition continued until 1975, when the professions became subject to anti-trust laws. By then, widespread abuse of insurance and Medicare policies were effectively preventing price competition among physicians. The careful control of the physician supply during the last century also restrained competition among physicians.

1920-1933: The XVIIIth Amendment and Alcohol Prohibition

Alcohol prohibition is mentioned here only to contrast it with narcotics prohibition, and to compare the implications for healthcare costs. Alcohol, when abused, is certainly as addictive and injurious to health as the narcotics that are still criminalized under federal and state laws.

Suppose hypothetically that Congress never had the temporary lapse of insanity that resulted in the repeal of alcohol prohibition. Suppose we treated alcohol like narcotics, and all alcohol addicts, "recreational users" and even "social drinkers" had to go to a doctor and get a prescription for alcohol every six months. What effect do you think that would have on healthcare costs? How would it affect crowding and wait times in clinic waiting rooms? How would it affect the costs of law enforcement, and our judicial and penal systems? What sort of bootlegging, smuggling and gangsterism would be reported in the daily news? What would the impact be on the cost, selection, and availability of alcoholic beverages? Most importantly, do you think alcohol prohibition would result in a reduction in alcohol abuse sufficient to justify all the unintended consequences?

1929 & 1939: Blue Cross Blue Shield Insurance is Founded

Blue Cross hospitalization insurance was essentially created and promoted by hospitals to ensure their bills got paid. It originated in 1929 at Baylor University's healthcare facilities in Dallas, and the first plan guaranteed up to 21 days of hospitalization per year for teachers, for $6 a year. In ensuing decades, it was extended to other groups and to all states. Official affiliation with the AHA (American Hospital Association) ended in 1972.

The first Blue Shield plan to cover physician services originated in California in 1939. It was essentially created and promoted by physicians as a means of ensuring their bills got paid. Because they were embraced and promoted by hospitals and doctors early on, Blue Cross and Blue Shield became the dominant medical insurers in America within a few decades. Blue Shield merged with Blue Cross in 1982 to form the Blue Cross and Blue Shield (BCBS) Association, an affiliated group of 38 independent, community-based and locally operated insurance companies that together serve all 50 states. Nearly 100 million Americans are currently covered by the various BCBS insurers.

It is important to note that, although promoted by doctors and hospitals, BCBS did not originate as a private for-profit insurance company. Rather, it originated as a non-profit organization with the mission of ensuring members of the community would be able to pay their doctor and hospital bills. BCBS organizations were tax exempt as social welfare plans until the Tax Reform Act of 1986. Thereafter, they were subject to federal taxation, but entitled to special tax benefits. Since 1994, the BCBS Association has allowed licensees to be for-profit corporations, although some are still registered as non-profit organizations [41].

Its non-profit, community-oriented origins and mission have shaped BCBS policies. Early on, most plans practiced "community rating" (all enrollees paid similar premiums, regardless of health status, based on the average healthcare costs of people in the community); and all applicants were accepted, regardless of pre-existing conditions ("guaranteed issue"). Such altruistic practices facilitated the BCBS goal of maximum coverage, but they also incentivized over-use of services, and decreased incentives for risk reduction. For instance, as healthcare costs and premium costs increased, guaranteed issue encouraged patients to wait until they got sick to buy insurance. In recent decades, as healthcare costs have escalated, it has become increasingly difficult for such policies to remain financially viable.

1932: The AAMC Recommends Reducing the Physician Supply

In 1932 the Association of American Medical Colleges' Commission on Medical Education again warned of a surplus of physicians, based on studies of population needs [32]. Despite this recommendation, the ratio of physicians to population continued to increase. What's important to point out here is that, despite periodic warnings by august commissions of a dire surplus or shortage of physicians, *there have never been enough medical school seats to accommodate the number of qualified applicants.* A substantial artificial barrier to entry for aspirants to the medical profession has been consistently maintained.

1938-1951: The Durham-Humphrey Amendment [29, 30, 31]

Prior to 1914 there were no federal laws to prohibit you from obtaining any medication without a doctor's prescription. The 1914 Harrison Narcotics Act (see above) required a prescription for narcotics. Subsequent legislation beginning with the 1938 U.S. Food, Drug, and Cosmetic Act, and culminating in the Durham-Humphrey Amendment of 1951, expanded the prescription requirement to any drug that is habit forming or "potentially harmful."

It is important to note that *everything under the sun* is "potentially harmful." Take, for example, the two most vital substances for our existence: oxygen and water. If you breathe 100% oxygen for longer than 24 hours, it will cause your lungs to become inflamed and fill up with fluid, and you will die. Or if you sit by your kitchen sink and drink one glass of water every 3 minutes, within an hour or so, your brain will swell up from absorbing excess water, causing seizures, coma and probably death. So the "potentially harmful" requirement is a license for bureaucrats to potentially ban *anything* they think you're too stupid to handle, including oxygen and water.

Interestingly, these laws do not seem to have been motivated by any problem with patients mismanaging their medications or accidently poisoning or overdosing themselves [39]. The laws appear to have been partly motivated by public outrage following the "Elixir Sulfanilamide disaster." In that disaster, an unscrupulous drug company, *with no prior safety testing*, marketed an elixir for common maladies that contained diethylene glycol, a well-known poison. Over 100 people, many of them children, died before Elixer Sulfanilamide could be removed from the market.

These laws addressed a real need for improved drug testing and labeling, and were clearly intended to improve public safety. Notwithstanding, the Durham-Humphrey Amendment is a classic example of the law of unintended effects. While it intended neither to deprive Americans of our right to manage our own healthcare, nor to increase the cost of healthcare, those have been significant enduring effects.

The laws preceding the Durham-Humphrey Amendment mandated labeling of all medications, but resulted in controversy regarding who was responsible for the labeling. One major motivation for the Durham-Humphrey Amendment was to settle that controversy. All medications would be classified into two groups: "OTC" (over the counter) drugs, to be labeled by the manufacturer; and "Legend" drugs, which the prescribing physician would be responsible for labeling (or providing the necessary patient information). Of course, the only way to require the physician to provide such information would be to require the patient to see a physician to obtain the medication!

The assumption that patients needed directions for use led to the problem of who would be responsible for providing such directions. By assigning this responsibility to physicians (clearly with the blessing of the AMA), Congress created a situation in which patients were required to visit physicians to obtain that information before they could obtain the medications. That might be helpful, assuming doctors actually provided such information, but couldn't we get it more conveniently from a pharmacist, or on the Internet? To further put this into perspective, note that far more people die every year from complications of obesity than ever died because of drug misinformation. Should we be required by law to visit a nutritionist and get prescriptions for our food and beverages, to ensure we eat a healthy diet?

The preceding interpretation of motivations is debatable. Some would claim that "elitist" special interests were a major driver of the Durham-Humphrey Amendment. But regardless of its motivations, the Durham-Humphrey Amendment marks the absolute triumph of elitism in American medicine. No matter how well educated, the ordinary person was no longer allowed to manage his or her own healthcare. A state-certified expert must be consulted for access to most medications. Unfortunately, laws are rarely repealed simply because they don't accomplish the intended effect… especially once powerful special interests become addicted to the *unintended* effects.

Elitism issues aside, the Durham-Humphrey Amendment is an excellent example of the laws of unintended effects and incentives (see Chapter 3):

1. Americans were deprived of the right to manage their own healthcare, and patients were *incentivized to become more dependent on their doctors and consult them more often.*

2. Doctors' incomes and net healthcare costs increased as patients were *incentivized to visit doctors more often.*

3. Doctors were *incentivized to prescribe more chronic medications*, because the requirement for refills would ensure a steady stream of return visits for any patient on a chronic medication.

4. Pharmaceutical companies were *incentivized to market directly to physicians*, since they now controlled drug purchases. Over time, such marketing evolved into an entirely-too-cozy (and often outright unethical) relationship, where the manufacturers of high-priced new drugs used incentives ranging from mini-skirted, college-fresh "drug representatives" bearing free donuts, to all-expense-paid "continuing education events" at expensive resorts.

5. Once they realized they controlled a money-spigot for the drug companies, many physicians realized they could double their benefit by investing in drug company stocks. Owning stock in the drug companies further incentivized physicians to prescribe more of the newest, most expensive drugs.

6. The AMA was incentivized to evolve from a staunch promoter of physician professionalism and quality care into a lackey of special interests, as revenue from pharmaceutical companies (for ads in AMA journals and fees for physician mailing lists) skyrocketed, and soon dwarfed AMA revenue from physician membership dues.

7. Because prescription drugs are harder to get, patients are incentivized to perceive them as "more powerful" or "more effective" than OTC medications. To this day, the "common cold" (viral upper respiratory infection) is one of the two most frequent reasons for physician visits, *even though no prescription medication is more beneficial than OTC remedies.* Nonetheless, most patients leave the doctor's office with a prescription. They get better a day or two later, which would have happened regardless, as the infection runs its course. Nonetheless, their belief that the doctor visit and medication helped is reinforced, resulting in a return visit the next time they catch a cold.

Let's re-visit Joe, the mechanic, one last time. Motor vehicle accidents on America's highways claim approximately the same number of lives every year as suicide and homicide combined. Some of those horrible accidents are due to mechanical failures resulting from improper maintenance or repairs. Suppose Congress decided to divide all auto parts into two categories: OTC parts, safe for car owners to buy and install themselves; and "Legend" parts — those critical to car safety, like brake pads or steering components.

No longer can you go to AutoZone and get whatever you need to fix your car. To get any "safety-critical" part, you first have to get an appointment with a licensed auto mechanic, and get a prescription to take to AutoZone. How would that affect the cost of auto maintenance in America? How much would it improve auto maintenance and safety in America? Certainly it would be great news for licensed mechanics. Maybe not so good for America on the whole.

1945: World War II and the Post-War Era

There is no fundamental reason why employers should be involved in health insurance; it just increases complexity and costs, and reduces plan portability. The practice gained traction during World War II, when employers were prohibited by wartime price controls from competing for employees by raising wages. Consequently, they substituted fringe benefits such as paid health and life insurance.

The post-war economic boom brought prosperity, and the big industrial manufacturers were flush with profits. Consequently the unions, at the peak of their power, were able to demand and get generous fringe benefits. Those benefits often included employer-paid health insurance. The most important and enduring incentive however is likely the federal tax exemption: employer-provided health insurance premiums are exempt from federal income tax. Individually purchased insurance is not tax-exempt.

Check any dictionary, and you will note the purpose of insurance is to pay "a guaranteed and known small loss to prevent a large, possibly devastating loss"

[11]. Using insurance to pay for a flu vaccine or a routine doctor visit is akin to using auto insurance to pay for a flat tire repair or an oil change. It is fundamentally inefficient because (a) it introduces a third profit-seeking, resource-using entity into every transaction; (b) it complicates every transaction; and most importantly, (c) it removes responsibility for payment from the consumer, thereby removing the consumer's incentive to bargain-shop and economize. Even worse for doctor-patient relationships, it makes the *real customer* (the entity that must be pleased to obtain payment) not the patient, but the insurer.

Contrary to the fundamental purpose of insurance, post-war employer-paid insurance plans often included coverage for expenses such as office visits, tests and minor medical procedures. That made it much more appealing as a form of compensation, because then it could be used for routine expenses. Employers didn't mind because coverage for office visits didn't cost much (healthcare was still only about 4.5% of GDP in 1950). Insurance companies certainly didn't mind because, big expense or small, they always got their middleman cut.

In effect, federal incentives caused "medical insurance" to evolve from real insurance into a form of tax-exempt compensation for ordinary expenses. This not only directly increases the costs of financing healthcare, but has resulted in numerous other unintended consequences and perverse incentives that contribute to skyrocketing healthcare costs, as we discuss elsewhere.

1950-Present: The Relentless Escalation of Healthcare Costs

U.S. Health Care Costs in Dollars and as a Percentage of GDP [8]

Year	Total Costs	% of GDP
1950	$12.7 billion	4.5%
1965	$40 billion	6%
1980	$230 billion	9%
2000	$1.2 *trillion*	14%
2009	$2.6 *trillion*	17.3%

When federal policy began promoting widespread abuse of health insurance during World War II, healthcare was less than 5% of GDP. When Medicare was created by Congress in 1965, healthcare was 6% of GDP. When Medicare and Medicaid started price controls and central bureaucratic management policies in the early 1980s, healthcare was 9% of GDP. Today, it is rapidly approaching 18% of GDP. How long can we afford to continue the Medicare/Medicaid/PPACA approach to "controlling costs" in healthcare?

1950-1965: Doctors Find the Insurance Cookie-Jar

In the post-war years, due to the widespread misuse of health insurance, the payers of medical services became increasingly disconnected from the consumers of those services. Doctors soon discovered that, although a patient might complain about $50 for an office visit, they could send a bill for $250 to the patient's insurance company, and oddly enough, the insurance company would usually pay without question. So they started doing that more often. Who could blame them? Patients didn't mind their doctors buying big new mansions next to their bankers — as long as someone else was footing the bill.

1958-1959: The Surgeon General Warns of a Physician Shortage

In 1958, the Surgeon General's office issued the Bayne-Jones report, followed by the Bane report in 1959 [32]. These reports predicted a looming shortage of physicians and recommended constructing new medical schools and increasing enrollment for existing schools. This resulted in congressional action to increase the physician supply in the 1960s. While such actions present the illusion of medical school enrollment adapting to America's needs, the truth remains: *there have never been nearly enough medical school seats to accommodate the number of qualified applicants.*

1962: The Kefauver-Harris Drug Amendments

Thalidomide was a new medication for sleep and nausea that caused thousands of severe birth defects in Europe in the 1950's. It was not marketed in the U.S. because of FDA proof-of-safety regulations already in place at that time. Nonetheless, the shocking photographs of children with "flippers" in place of arms and legs evoked a strong emotional reaction in the U.S., and aroused public support for stronger drug laws. Congress's reaction was the Kefauver-Harris Drug Amendments.

Previous laws already required proof of safety for new drugs. Now drug makers would also be required to prove the *effectiveness* of new drugs before they could be marketed. That sounds reasonable enough. Unfortunately, as you will see, it has had significant adverse unintended consequences.

Traditionally, new drugs were formulated based on theoretical reasoning or testing by scientists or physicians. Drugs that appeared to affect a specific condition were tested inexpensively on small groups of people or animals. The final determination of effectiveness occurred over many years, as new drugs were tried on many real patients in the real world.

Keep in mind that laws mandating proof of *safety* were already in place, working effectively at the time of the Kefauver-Harris amendments. Proving efficacy is much more difficult, expensive and time-consuming than proving safety. The Kefauver-Harris amendments have had all the following negative effects:

1. Due to the enormous costs and long time required to conduct large-scale human trials that prove efficacy, only very large or well-funded pharmaceutical companies are now able to field new drugs.

2. Consequently, new options for treatment of difficult diseases have declined. Because of the enormous investment required, drug companies tend to develop new drugs for only the most common diseases (so they have a large market) or the most lethal diseases (so patients are willing to pay a fortune).

3. Many beneficial effects of drugs that fail initial efficacy testing will never be discovered. It is a truism that new drugs often end up being most beneficial for uses entirely unanticipated when they are introduced. For example, aspirin was invented and marketed by the Bayer Company in the 1890s as an analgesic. It wasn't until 50 years later that it was discovered to prevent heart attacks and strokes.

4. A new drug should be evaluated based on how it compares with pre-existing treatments for its intended use. But the FDA doesn't mandate such comparisons; it only requires proof that a new drug works *better than nothing*! That allows drug companies to market new drugs as "effective" when they are actually *less effective* than older generic medications.

5. The international competitiveness and pre-eminence of U.S. drug and device manufacturers has been seriously eroded by the FDA's aggressive over-regulation that inhibits innovation and investment in new drugs and devices.

In reality, the effectiveness and potential uses of a new drug or device can only be determined by doctors and patients in the real world over a long time. What might be helpful, instead of mandating proof of efficacy, would be to:

1. Require drug makers to label their drugs, stating plainly what benefits have or have not been proven, and

2. Empower the FDA to study the available evidence and approve (or proscribe) manufacturers' efficacy claims.

We are beginning to see a pattern here:

a) Some high-profile event or catastrophe arouses public emotions and demand for government response. Or perhaps it just arouses come congressperson's desire to play hero.

b) Congress, acting under arbitrary time pressure and with high ignorance regarding the complex systems under regulation, overreacts with massive and expensive legislation.

c) An onslaught of new regulations erodes the freedoms of both individuals and corporations, while escalating complexity and costs throughout the system.

d) It often becomes obvious in hindsight that the triggering event was a statistical fluke that would likely have never recurred, or that it was already addressed by existing laws, if they had only been adequately enforced.

e) It often becomes obvious in hindsight that far simpler legislation would have adequately addressed the problem; and that the negative unintended consequences and perverse incentives far outweigh any benefit of the legislation.

f) By then, bureaucracies, businesses, special interests, and even the public have become adapted and addicted to the perverse collateral "benefits" of counterproductive legislation. Inertia and benefits for powerful special interest groups work against change, making it difficult to repeal even the most harmful legislation.

New drug development declined significantly after 1962, and the wait for new life-saving drugs to come on the market had increased to more than a decade by the end of the 1970s. Today it costs up to *a billion dollars* and takes 12-15 years to bring a new drug to market.

1963-1967: Congressional Action Increases the Supply of Physicians

In 1963, the Health Professions Education Assistance Act provided funds for new Medical school construction to increase the supply of physicians. This action was at least partly a response to the Bayne-Jones (1958) and Bane (1959) reports mentioned above, and was supported by succeeding reports, including the Coggeshall report to the AAMC in 1965, which stated "more physicians must be trained as quickly as possible" [32]. In 1967, the President's National Advisory Committee on Health Manpower called for rapid increases in medical school enrollment. By 1968, both the AAMC (Association of American Medical Colleges) and the AMA expressed commitment to medical school expansion.

It is noteworthy, however, that there have never been enough medical school slots to accommodate the number of young people wanting to enter the profession. In 1975, only about one in five qualified applicants was being admitted. In more recent decades the figure has risen to 40-50% of qualified applicants. This rise likely reflects a combination of more medical schools and lower application rates. Lower application rates likely reflect a relative decline in the pay, prestige and opportunities of physicians in recent years. In any event, it is obvious that artificial barriers to entry into the medical profession have consistently prevented the law of supply and demand from bringing down physician fees, as it would in a less regulated marketplace.

1966: Medicare and the Dawn of a New Age

In 1966, when Medicare appeared on the scene, insurance abuse was already spreading like kudzu, but healthcare costs still only accounted for about 6% of GDP. Initially, Medicare functioned much like any other insurance company, albeit one created by the federal government explicitly for seniors (more precisely, for Social Security beneficiaries). Since seniors are mostly retired and have time to vote, and because many were recently retired from jobs that provided medical "insurance" that covered minor expenses such as office visits, Congress enshrined that fundamental abuse of insurance in Medicare.

Initially Medicare, like private insurance companies at the time, generally paid whatever claims doctors submitted, without questioning. How could they question the bills? With no standardized terminology for medical billing, Medicare had no idea what the items on the bills represented or how much they were worth. Consequently, many doctors, mindless of the long-term ramifications, routinely plundered the Medicare cookie jar, just as they did with private insurance. Big mistake.

If it weren't for Medicare, the fundamental problem of insurance abuse (and the resulting consumer-payer disconnect) might have been corrected by free-market forces. With escalating costs, insurance companies would have been forced to increase premiums dramatically for policies with comprehensive coverage, thus forcing most patients back to catastrophic coverage. Patients paying out of pocket for most services would be incentivized to conserve and comparison shop, thus restoring the consumer-payer connection. Similarly, doctors would be incentivized to compete on price and quality, just like other service providers.

Competition in the healthcare market would have been greatly facilitated by the 1975 court victory of the FTC over the AMA, which ended the AMA's promulgation of "usual and customary" fees and its prohibition of physician advertising and solicitation (see later in this chapter). Unfortunately, Medicare took a different approach, and we are all still suffering the multitudinous unintended consequences.

1970s: The Decline of the AMA and "Organized Medicine"

The AMA had long been a strong voice on behalf of American physicians and initially opposed Medicare. That stance lasted until they began to share in the financial benefits of the new program. AMA membership peaked around 1963, two years before Congress legislated Medicare, at 71% of practicing physicians. By 1971, membership had declined to about 63% of practicing physicians, and has continued to decline.

In 1983, the AMA contracted with HCFA (the Health Care Financing Administration) to provide the "CPT codes" used by Medicare and Medicaid (and subsequently by private insurance) to "chain" physicians to menus of services reimbursed according to fixed fee schedules. In recent years, AMA income from licensing fees (for these codes, and sales of printed materials and software to help physicians cope with them) has exceeded physician membership dues. Membership is now down to approximately 17% of practicing physicians, reflecting the fact that most physicians no longer regard the AMA as a valid representative of the medical profession.

At this point, the AMA is heavily invested in, and financially addicted to, our current exorbitantly inefficient system. Consequently, it is happy to trot out white-coated "representatives of Organized Medicine" to support reactionary attempts, such as the PPACA, to sustain and expand the current system.

1974: The Employee Retirement Income Security Act (ERISA)

This act focused on the regulation of employer-provided pension plans, but actually liberated employer-provided health insurance. In a nutshell, it permitted employers to self-ensure — essentially to become health insurance companies for their employees. Today, many large companies self-ensure. Since they are not regulated as insurance companies, however, such employers have had tremendous freedom with regard to what providers and services are covered, and how much to charge employees for premiums. They also have not been required, unlike insurance companies, to maintain cash reserves in proportion to the amount of risk covered.

Mid-1970s to Mid-1980s: The Malpractice Insurance Crises

Inevitably, physicians' high incomes combined with their omnipresence during medical tragedies conspired to make them attractive targets for liability lawsuits. In the mid-1970s, doctors experienced a crisis of malpractice insurance availability. Due to the increasing number and amount of malpractice awards, many malpractice insurers abandoned the market, leaving doctors unable to obtain insurance at any price. In response, physician organizations created non-profit, physician-owned "mutual" insurance companies, such as State Volunteer Mutual Insurance Company.

In the mid-1980s, the high rate of malpractice lawsuits and increasing size of awards led to a crisis of insurance affordability. Even non-profit mutual insurance companies must cover their costs. Some medical specialties (e.g., obstetrics and neurosurgery) are particularly prone to malpractice suits, resulting in astronomical premiums. In states where it was legal to do so, some physicians "went bare," dropping malpractice insurance altogether. That resulted in a thriving market among accountants, attorneys and financial planners for other types of "asset protection services" to help physicians shield their assets from court judgments.

Ultimately, doctors' and hospitals' malpractice insurance premiums and malpractice suit defense and award costs end up being paid by patients and taxpayers. However, the direct costs of malpractice insurance are only the tip of the iceberg. Due to widespread (and well-justified) malpractice paranoia, virtually all doctors now practice "defensive medicine" to some degree. Many tests and treatments are ordered that might not be medically necessary or effective, but help shield doctors from accusations of insufficient diligence when, as often happens with even the best of care, patients have bad outcomes. We'll examine these costs again later.

1980s-1990s: Medicare Tightens the Screws

Soon after Medicare was introduced, it became apparent that costs were increasing much more rapidly than Congress had projected. By now, that shouldn't surprise you. Why not order every test in the book and use the most expensive treatments? Patients don't care, as long as someone else is paying most of the charges;

and doctors don't want to risk a $10,000,000 lawsuit for overlooking an unlikely diagnosis.

Something had to be done. Congress should have addressed the root causes, including insurance abuse and the resulting consumer-payer disconnect, high barriers to entry, out-of-control malpractice litigation, and unwise restriction of patients' self-care options. Instead, Congress radically compounded the problem by imposing price controls on all doctors and hospitals participating in the Medicare program. This occurred incrementally, primarily during the period from 1983 through 1992.

Most economists agree that price controls are a bad idea. They cause widespread mismatches between supply and demand, and that results in widespread shortages, surpluses, and rationing. Unfortunately, price controls remain the kneejerk reaction of most politicians when confronted with out-of-control inflation.

Because healthcare is complex, involving thousands of procedures, drugs and devices, all affected by ongoing research and innovation, fixing prices wasn't as simple as setting the price of gasoline. Consequently, many healthcare organizations now devote more effort to meeting (and gaming) Medicare's payment rules and regulations, than to actual patient care. As any economist would have predicted, efficiency has been going down, and costs have continued to rise much faster than inflation.

If the current oppressive system of price controls and bureaucratic regulation had been applied in a single blow, both patients and physicians would certainly have stood up in unison and screamed "NO

WAY." It is only because the current regulations were applied incrementally over decades, each step seeming at least tolerable, that we have allowed our healthcare system to reach its current over-priced, inefficient, dysfunctional state.

1980: Physician Supply Has Markedly Increased and Authorities Warn of a Doctor Surplus

By 1982 the number of U.S. medical schools had increased to 127, up from 89 schools in 1972. Combined with increased enrollment in existing schools, this resulted in a doubling of the number of medical school graduates [32].

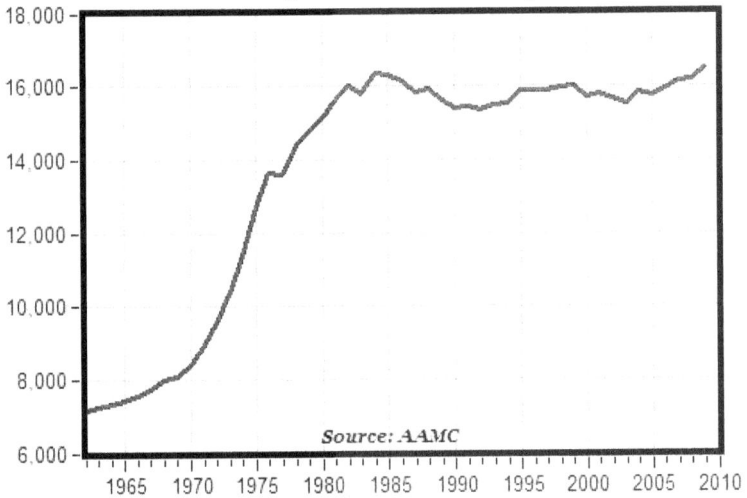

As you can see from the above graph, the annual number of medical school graduates increased dramatically because of congressional action in the mid-60s, combined with a broad-based concern among both private and government organizations related to physician education and supply.

"In 1980, the Graduate Medical Education National Advisory Committee (GMENAC) reported (based upon the number of physicians needed to provide "necessary and appropriate" services) that a surplus of 70,000 physicians would be likely by the year 2000… With the promotion of tightly controlled managed care in the early 1990s, many groups reaffirmed the belief that the nation was facing a surplus. The national Council on Graduate Medical Education (COGME), the National Academy of Science's Institute of Medicine (IOM), the Pew Health Professions Commission, the AAMC, the AMA and other national physician associations expressed concerns about an impending potential surplus of physicians" [32].

The preceding paragraph reveals the sort of economic nonsense that prevails in mainstream healthcare policy-making. Implicit in the above recommendations is the warped notion that having "too many physicians" will further drive up healthcare costs. In our current dysfunctional system, where all any doctor has to do is get in-network with the top insurance companies and then "churn patients" to generate a $250,000 income, that may be true. But in a free market, where all the people with the intelligence and desire to become doctors were allowed to do so, and patients were free to pick their doctors, drugs and devices based on price and preference, the effect would be quite different. As a point of comparison, to emphasize the absurdity of national healthcare policy, can you imagine august national commissions warning Congress of "an impending potential surplus" of short-order cooks, carpenters, accountants or plumbers?

Similar nonsense has prevailed in policies and legislation regarding hospitals. Instead of allowing hospitals to compete wherever they want, some states have enacted legislation requiring a "certificate of need" before a new hospital can be constructed! Can you imagine how affordable and available groceries and building supplies would be if federal bureaucracies set all the prices and states required a "certificate of need" before a new supermarket or Home Depot was allowed to open in your neighborhood?

1985: The Consolidated Omnibus Budget Reconciliation Act (COBRA)

This act addressed the widespread problem of employees losing their insurance when they left an employer. It gave employees the right to remain on their employer's group plan for up to 18 months, *if they paid 102% of the premium*. By this time, healthcare (and its insurance) had become quite expensive. Since employers typically paid 75% of the premiums, under COBRA a newly unemployed person was confronted with a four-fold increase in their monthly insurance premium, on top of a sudden loss of income. Consequently, in general only unhealthy people with high medical expenses take advantage of COBRA. Though not an affordable solution for between-job insurance for most people, COBRA at least provided a bridge between jobs for those who could afford it.

For our purposes here, COBRA marks the beginning of the federal regulatory "takeover" of the medical insurance industry that we will see consummated in the 2011 PPACA (Obamacare). Unfortunately, like so much legislation that preceded and followed them, these acts do not address the fundamental problems. They are only shortsighted symptomatic Band-Aids, with more adverse unintended consequences than benefits.

1990-Present: The Steady Decline in Small Practices

As detailed in the charts and graphs below, and in the stories of thousands of doctors all over America, solo and small-group physician practices are disappearing. Hospitals and corporations are buying up practices, and the remaining physician-owned practices are increasingly large multi-physician and multi-specialty practices in larger towns and cities. Solo and small physician groups can simply no longer afford the coders, billing and insurance specialists, lawyers, accountants, and "compliance specialists" required to survive in our current system.

Percentage of Family Physicians in Solo and 2-Physician Practices

	1980	1997
Solo Practice	54%	25%
2-Physician Practice	14%	8%

As shown in the chart above, between 1980 and 1997 the percentage of family physicians in solo and 2-doctor groups declined by one-half [46].

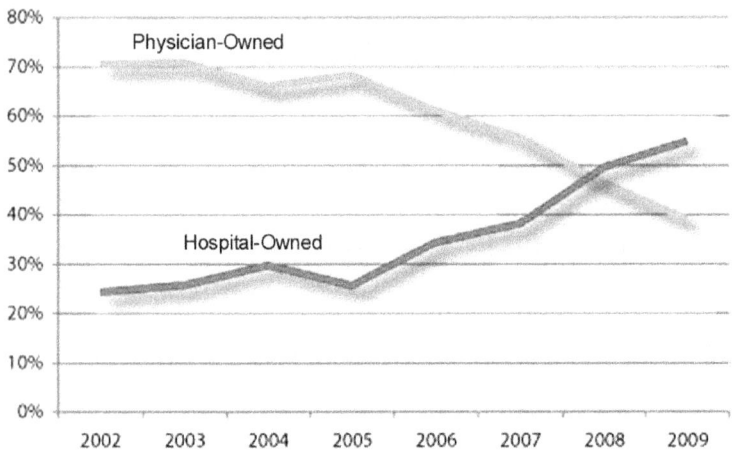

Percentage of Practices Owned by Physicians and Hospitals

The graph above shows a precipitous decline in physician ownership of practices in the past decade. (Data from the Physician Compensation and Production Survey, Medical Group Management Association, 2002-2009.)

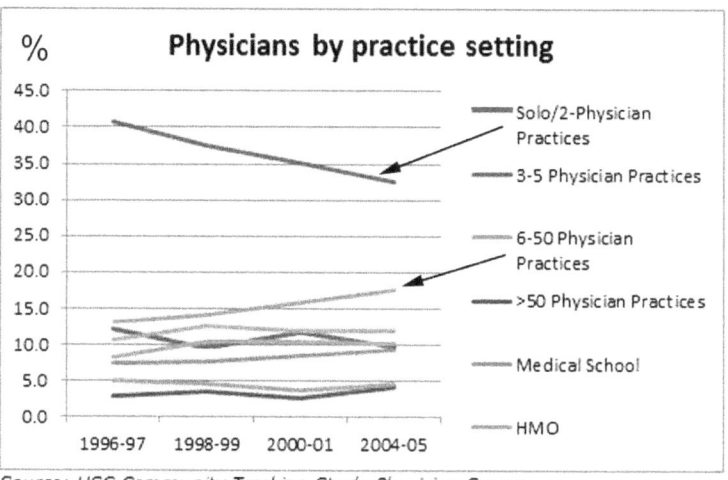

Source: HSC Community Tracking Study Physician Survey

The top two lines of this graph show a steep decline in solo and 2-physician practices from 1996 to 2005, accompanied by a rise in groups with 6-50 physicians, as physicians coalesce into larger practices.

Are we wise to continue the policies that make it impossible for solo and small-group practices to survive?

1990s: A Glut of Doctors?

In 1994, COGME (the Committee on Graduate Medical Education) reported to Congress and the Secretary of Health and Human Services, "In a managed care dominated health system, the Bureau of Health Professions projects a year 2000 shortage of 35,000 generalist physicians and a surplus of 115,000 specialist physicians." Consequently, COGME recommended a 25% reduction in medical school graduates. Other authoritative organizations, including the Pew Commission, the Institute of Medicine, and the AAMC warned of an impending surplus of physicians in the 1990s and recommended decreased medical school enrollment and/or reduction of public funds for medical education.

In response, the number of graduates from U.S. medical schools remained stable between 1980 and 2005. However, due to the increase in medical school enrollment in the '60s and '70s, the physician supply, in both relative and absolute terms, continued to increase, from 202 physicians per 100,000 people in 1980 to 276 per 100,000 in 2000.

Are we really threatened with a surplus of physicians? Have you ever encountered an unemployed physician? When was the last time a doctor offered to cut you a deal to get your business? Yet we still periodically hear apocalyptic warnings of a dire physician surplus, based on the warped economic theory that an increase in supply will make prices go up.

1996: The Health Insurance Portability and Accountability Act (HIPAA)

This act places the following requirements on group insurance providers, including self-ensuring employers:

1. It mandates "guaranteed issue" (every member of the group must be eligible for coverage).
2. It sets limits and restrictions on waiting periods for pre-existing conditions.

3. It prohibits charging higher premiums to individuals within a group based on individual health status.

Although it pretends in its title to promote insurance portability, this act actually did the opposite. Some employers had previously purchased individual insurance for their employees, which the employees could continue when they left the company. HIPPAA has been interpreted, however, as mandating that only group insurance can be tax-exempt. Consequently, all employer-provided insurance became group insurance, which usually terminates when an employee leaves the group.

HIPPA is actually most notorious among healthcare businesses and professionals for its strict regulation of the handling of patient medical records. The primary intent of these regulations is to ensure the privacy of patient health records. The HIPAA privacy regulations seem (in my opinion) to be quite reasonable, and in general they reflect policies already prevailing at many healthcare organizations at the time. Nonetheless, because the privacy regulations are vaguely written, they have been subject to variable interpretation. Consequently, they have generated widespread anxiety and resentment among doctors, and have spawned a minor industry of literature, software and consulting targeted at "HIPPA compliance."

2003: A Jury Awards $58,600,000 in a Malpractice Case

In 2003, a jury in Connecticut ordered Dr. Richard Viscarello to pay $58.6 million in damages to the parents of a child born with cerebral palsy. This represented a new high in the long-term trend toward larger malpractice awards [33].

Several states have moved to mitigate this trend in recent years. In 2003, the Texas legislature passed laws that capped non-economic damages at $250,000 for individual physicians and $500,000 for medical institutions. This law has apparently resulted in a significant increase in the number of physicians obtaining licensure in Texas. The law also increased the proportion of "high risk" specialists in the state. For example, the number of rural obstetricians increased by 27% and the number of orthopedic surgeons by 15%.

2011: The PPACA Masquerades as Healthcare Reform

The Patient Protection and Affordable Care Act of 2011 is not healthcare reform. It is, in fact, quite conservative. Any objective reading of recent history and the provisions of the law can lead to only one conclusion: the PPACA is a reactionary attempt to conserve and expand the very policies that created our current healthcare crisis. That is the subject of the next chapter.

Chapter 5
The PPACA (Obamacare) — Problems and Solutions

The Patient Protection and Affordable Care Act of 2011 (the PPACA, aka Obamacare) is not reform at all. Rather, it is a reactionary attempt to conserve and expand the same policies that created our current healthcare crisis, as will be described in this chapter. Consequently, we can confidently predict that the PPACA will become harder to defend as time passes. Without real reform, healthcare costs will almost certainly continue to climb from their current 18% of GDP toward 25%. As that happens, we can also expect that:

1. Our general prosperity and productivity will decline as even more resources are consumed by our dysfunctional healthcare system.

2. Healthcare will become increasingly unaffordable and inconvenient for the middle class and poor alike. This will likely result in a distinctly two-tiered system.

3. Work in the healthcare system will become increasingly unpleasant, as workers are increasingly subjected to perverse incentives, and prevented from focusing on their true missions.

4. We will become less competitive in the international marketplace because our economy will be paying over $10,000 for every family member of every employee for healthcare.

Those costs are inevitably included in the prices of our goods and services.

It should be noted that the PPACA is an enabling act that sets up the infrastructure for later implementation by some 159 new bureaucracies. Many important details are not specified in the law itself, but will be dictated by these new bureaucracies, insulated from feedback at the ballot box.

Let's examine the problems of the PPACA, and discuss some possible solutions.

Problem 1: The PPACA perpetuates and expands Medicare's counterproductive medical price controls and central bureaucratic "management" policies. As summarized by the law of supply and demand, fluid price agreements *within* the marketplace can efficiently match supplies of goods and services to patient needs and preferences. Price controls, in contrast, inevitably lead to all sorts of perverse incentives and inefficient behaviors throughout the system. Providers are incentivized to game the system instead of pleasing patients.

Solution: Get rid of price controls and allow healthcare providers to compete based on quality, reputation and price. The fact that many will consider *this* a radical idea only reveals how disconnected from both economic reality and American ideals our healthcare system has become.

Problem 2: In response to the variability in quality among hospitals, schemes will be implemented to tie reimbursement to measures of quality. History demonstrates, however, that any bureaucratically contrived compensation system will have questionable validity and effectiveness. Correspondingly, the resulting economic gains will certainly be more than offset by stakeholders "gaming" the system, and a slew of new adverse unintended effects will be created.

For example, suppose physician compensation is tied to successful health outcomes. Say a doctor receives $2000 a year for treating a patient who is compliant with their plan, quits smoking, comes in for preventative care, loses weight, and keeps their blood pressure and cholesterol down. Now suppose that same doctor receives only $500 a year for treating a non-compliant patient, because that patient's blood pressure and cholesterol are out of control. Will the doctor make daily calls to the non-compliant patient, coaxing them to come in for their counseling and checkups? Far more likely, non-compliant patients will be neglected, while doctors and clinics focus on recruiting and retaining the better-paying patients.

Solution: As in any other industry, the people most qualified (actually, the *only people qualified*) to judge the quality of a product or service are its *consumers*. The most efficient way to give feedback to producers is for consumers to "vote with their wallets." In this regard, Congress should ban Medicare and discourage private insurance companies from creating contract "networks." Rather, patients should be free to spend their insurance or Medicare dollars with any doctor they choose. This would cost far less than the additional layers of bureaucracy to implement pools and networks as envisioned by PPACA, and would actually improve quality and patient satisfaction.

Problem 3: The PPACA proposes to fund expanded coverage partly by forcing employers to provide medical insurance. In an economy with ever-increasing worker mobility, fluctuating unemployment, and increased outsourcing of jobs to cheaper labor markets abroad, burdening employers with the cost of providing health insurance makes no more sense than forcing them to provide potato blight insurance or piano lessons!

Solution: Individually purchased medical insurance should be tax-favored (or not) the same as employer-provided insurance. Insurance policies should be portable across state lines. Incentives to expand coverage will be discussed in the next chapter.

Problem 4: The PPACA mandates that all qualified insurance plans provide *comprehensive* and *preventative* healthcare coverage. This is contrary to the basic definition of insurance. Using insurance to pay for a flu vaccine, a school physical or to treat poison ivy is akin to using insurance to buy groceries or to fill up your gas tank. It simply encourages over-spending, while greatly increasing costs of basic services by adding the costs of extra paperwork, money shuffling and reimbursement issues. Furthermore, by removing the consumer's role as payer, it removes the consumer's incentive to economize; and it incentivizes doctors and hospitals to please the insurers instead of patients.

Solution: Congress should encourage high-deductible insurance policies linked to HSAs (Health Savings Accounts; see* below). That would decrease overall costs and discourage over-utilization of primary care services, while encouraging individual accountability and retirement planning.

Presumably, part of the motivation for mandating first-dollar coverage for preventive care is to decrease total healthcare costs. Unfortunately, the evidence for net cost reductions from current preventive care recommendations is scant to non-existent. For example, after decades of oscillation, authorities have recently decided men should *not* get periodic PSA prostate cancer screening because it *increases* net costs, and does more harm than good.

In any event, patients and their doctors should be allowed to decide what screening they want, based on personal preferences and current evidence. According to the PPACA philosophy, what might be next? Government-mandated exercise, twice-daily flossing, and quarterly oil changes? Is that really the direction we want to be headed?

[*A Health Savings Account (HSA) is a savings account specifically for routine, out-of-pocket medical expenses. It is used in combination with a high-deductible insurance policy for unusual, big expenses (the true definition of insurance). The employer makes an automatic tax-free deposit to the HSA every pay period. Any money in the HSA not used for medical expenses remains in the account, accumulating interest tax-free. The money can be withdrawn for other purposes only by paying income tax plus a 20% penalty. After retirement, the money can be used for other purposes without penalty. A "Roth HSA" is funded with after-tax money, but accumulates interest tax-free.]

Problem 5: By prohibiting premium discounts for lifestyle factors (smoking excepted), the PPACA discourages personal responsibility for health outcomes, despite the fact that *more than half of all chronic disease and disability in the U.S. is attributable to individual lifestyle choices* (lack of exercise, overeating, poor food choices, smoking, excessive alcohol consumption, reckless driving, etc.) [8, 9]. This issue also strikes at the heart of the fairness issue: Why should people who choose healthy lifestyles be required to subsidize those who choose unhealthy lifestyles?

Solution: To discourage unhealthy or risky behavior, taxpayer-provided healthcare should be partially financed through targeted taxation of products and activities proven to contribute to disease and disability. Insurance companies should be *encouraged* to give discounts for healthy lifestyles. How is that different from auto insurance companies giving discounts for good driving records and safety education?

Problem 6: Health insurance reforms are needed to prevent specific abuses, and to increase insurance portability and continuity. Instead of addressing the underlying problems, the PPACA takes the same approach to the insurance industry that Medicare has taken toward doctors and hospitals, with spectacularly disastrous results. The PPACA imposes price controls on the insurance industry (preventing the Law of Supply and Demand and price signaling from functioning), mandates first-dollar coverage of routine expenses (defying the definition of insurance and perpetuating the consumer-payer disconnect), and prohibits price variation based on risk (again defying the definition of insurance and incentivizing unhealthy lifestyles).

By requiring all Americans to buy this over-priced non-insurance, the PPACA essentially converts America's private health insurance industry into a giant income-redistribution scheme. These mandates, combined with the expansion of Medicaid, funnel funds from healthy and middle or high-income healthcare consumers to unhealthy and low-income, unemployed, or disabled healthcare consumers.

To accomplish the same amount of income redistribution less clandestinely would require enormous new tax increases and entitlements. Such legislation would be political suicide for its authors. Cloaking this massive income redistribution in private insurance mandates allows it to be accomplished without explicit taxation or entitlements. The irony is that, in the long run, this scheme is going to make us all poorer, and *those who are poorest will suffer most.*

Solution: Congress should impose only the minimum insurance regulations needed to prevent egregious practices, to promote insurance policy portability and continuity, and to promote competition in the insurance industry. For example, insurers should be encouraged to provide policies that guarantee renewability, and that insure against rate increases when a patient develops chronic or expensive diseases in the future. Just as with life insurance, young or healthy people would be protected against rate increases when they get old or sick.

In general, Congress should abandon its delusion that it has the power to flaunt the fundamental laws of economics, or redefine the concept of insurance. Massive income redistribution schemes should not be disguised as "healthcare reform." Clearly, some amount of income redistribution will be required to ensure that even the poorest and least healthy Americans have access to healthcare. The net cost to American taxpayers will be far less with real healthcare reform that doesn't flaunt the basic laws of economics and quixotically attempt to redefine the concept of insurance.

Problem 7: The PPACA aspires to provide affordable healthcare to all Americans. But its policies contradict the fundamental laws of economics, and will therefore cause healthcare to become increasingly unaffordable for both the middleclass and poor alike.

Solution: To provide a medical "safety net" for all Americans, Congress or the states should provide vouchers so that those unable to afford healthcare can purchase it in the private market, much as "food stamp" recipients receive funds to spend, according to their preferences, in any grocery store. The federal takeover and management of our healthcare system to "control prices" and ensure availability of healthcare for all Americans makes no more sense than a federal takeover of our food industry to ensure adequate nutrition for all Americans. *That approach is what caused the problem.*

Problem 8: The PPACA guarantees escalating healthcare costs in the future by prohibiting "any annual or lifetime limit on coverage." There is virtually no limit to how much can be spent extending the life of a dying person another few weeks or months. For that matter, in a creative and entrepreneurial culture such as ours, if the PPACA isn't repealed there will soon be no limit on how much can be spent in one year to treat a typical teenager's acne!

In every industry there are trade-offs between quality and cost. How much would you pay for increased vehicle safety? Would you buy a $70,000 car because it is twice as safe as a $35,000 car? Would you pay $125,000 for a vehicle that is 10% safer than the $70,000 model? We make trade-offs like this every day; it's an integral part of any economic decision. It is irrational to think that such trade-offs can be ignored in healthcare without incurring astronomical costs.

No-limit or high-limit health insurance policies have long been available *for those wealthy enough to afford them*. Because insurance companies incur a high risk with such policies, and therefore higher average expenses, *they must charge relatively high premiums* for such policies if they want to stay in business. The PPACA mandate that insurance companies give no-limit policies to *everyone, while strictly limiting their ability to raise premiums*, simply defies the laws of mathematics — unless the real goal is to drive the insurance companies into bankruptcy.

This "Rolls-Royce insurance at Volkswagen prices" mandate is little different from the government decreeing that the housing industry must sell everyone a 20-room mansion for $100,000, or that our automakers must sell everyone an $80,000 luxury car for $10,000. Despite the popular appeal of such mandates, Congress does not have the power to legislate the laws of mathematics or perform Biblical miracles. This attempt to do so is bound to have serious adverse unintended consequences.

Solution: Congress should abandon its attempt to magically transform the health insurance industry into a golden goose. There will always be limits on what we can afford for a person's healthcare in any given year or lifetime. The ultimate clash between reality and this mandate to ignore it will inevitably result in serious unintended consequences.

Problem 9: The Congressional Budget Office estimated that the PPACA will cost roughly one trillion dollars over 10 years. That estimate includes only the government's direct costs. It ignores the enormous cost of America's healthcare system to implement the many thousands of pages of regulations that will ultimately result from the 2,700-page law. That is exactly the same mistake Congress has made in the past that resulted in Medicare's costs increasing more rapidly than anticipated.

It is very expensive to implement complex new rules and regulations throughout an industry. That requires imposing many new responsibilities on existing personnel, hiring many additional personnel, and a very long and expensive adjustment process that ends with substantially increased ongoing costs to accommodate the additional regulations. Even if all these new regulations only increase the current cost of healthcare by 5% (a modest estimate), that will translate to 1.1 trillion dollars of additional costs over the next 10 years. That *more than doubles* the CBO's cost estimate for the PPACA. The actual cost is likely to be even greater.

Solution: *The CBO should include reasonable estimates of the industry's implementation costs in any estimates of the cost of healthcare reform.* Then those estimates should be doubled or trebled, to account for the unintended consequences and perverse incentives that will inevitably result from the new regulations. Had that been done in the past, Congress's previous cost estimates would have been pretty much spot-on.

Problem 10: The PPACA discourages innovation and investment in health insurance by setting legal minimums on the medical loss ratio of 80% for individual and small group plans, and 85% for large group plans. The medical loss ratio (MLR) is the percent of income from policy premiums that is used to pay or reimburse healthcare costs or claims. In other words, if the minimum allowed medical loss ratio is 85%, then an insurance company's business costs and profits combined cannot exceed 15% of revenues. If medical losses are less than 85% of revenues, the difference cannot go to overhead or profit. It must be returned to policyholders as a rebate.

At first glance, this might sound like a reasonable way to enforce efficiency and cost cutting. But let's examine a typical scenario that might arise. Consider an insurance company that's comfortably achieving its 85% minimum MLR, with 8% overhead and 7% profit. Now suppose a bright young executive comes to the CEO and says, "Hey, Boss, there's a new treatment for hip arthritis that's just as effective as joint replacement, for a fraction of the cost. If we encourage our patients to use this new treatment, we could save $200 million a year on pay-outs, and double our profits!" The CEO replies, "Nice idea, Bob, but since we're already meeting our minimum MLR, we'd just have to rebate that $200,000,000 to our customers. Since our maximum overhead-plus-profits would then be only 15% of a pie that's $200 million smaller, our profits would actually go down! Why not take a nice, long coffee break, Bob — maybe play Angry Birds for a while?"

Limits on profits contradict the economic principle that risk-taking and innovation are driven by the profit incentive. For example, in a free market, if company A sees a way to improve operations that translates into increased profit, it will do so. Company B, offering the same service as A, will note the advantage and emulate A. It might find an even more efficient solution than A, thus enabling it to lower prices further to capture a larger share of the market.

While innovation allows companies to make larger profits in the short run, the net effect over time is improved efficiency and *lower prices* in the long run. That dynamic has driven constant improvements in our consumer products, while bringing down prices for many decades. *The PPACA prevents that from happening in healthcare and health insurance.* Though limiting profits may be superficially appealing to the economically illiterate, the long-term effect is to stifle innovation and competition, and inhibit price reductions.

Solution: By now, it should be apparent that there is no cure for the PPACA. It is simply 2700 pages of economic nonsense. The only "solution" for the PPACA is to make it a footnote in American History.

Chapter Summary

An examination of the PPACA in the light of fundamental principles of economics and human behavior shows it is unlikely to accomplish its stated goals. On the contrary, it is virtually certain to further ratchet up healthcare costs, with significant negative impacts on quality, accessibility and innovation. Ultimately, it will do great damage to our prosperity and international standing; and the people hurt most will be those it aspires to assist. The ignorance of its creators relative to the complexity of the healthcare system, combined with the large number of changes, guarantees its unintended consequences and perverse incentives will far outweigh its benefits over time.

Chapter 6
Unchaining American Healthcare

Americans' four largest expense categories are housing, food, transportation, and healthcare. Since 1950, our houses, food and cars have grown ever more efficient, abundant, and affordable. For example:

- In 1950 most families had one car, with hand-crank windows and no air-conditioning. Today, most families have one car for every licensed driver. Today's cars have automatic everything, air bags, anti-lock brakes, cruise control… and the list keeps growing.

- In 1950 the average middle-class home was 983 square feet, poorly insulated, had one bathroom, minimal appliances, and no air conditioning. Today's average middle-class home is 2100 square feet, has 2.5 bathrooms, central heating and cooling, and far more appliances — a mansion by comparison.

- In the 1950s a family had a single rotary-dial phone and one black-and-white television in the living room. There were no PCs, video game boxes, VCRs, or surround sound systems. Today, every family member has a cell phone starting, on average, at age 8. Each of those phones has more processing power than the computers that launched the first spacecraft to the moon. Every bedroom has a TV, and every family has a plasma or HD screen with surround sound. PCs are ubiquitous, and rapidly being replaced by tablets, and video games are as sophisticated as flight simulators.

- 60 years ago, most middle-class families could only afford steak one day per week, and under-nutrition among the poor was a significant problem. Today, even America's poor are seriously obese, and under-nutrition is virtually non-existent.

Why haven't we experienced a similar increase in the abundance and affordability of medical goods and services? During that same period, similar technological advances have occurred in healthcare, but medical services and devices have become dramatically more costly and inconvenient. Total healthcare costs have increased nearly four-fold relative to other categories, increasing from 4.5% to almost 18% of GDP since 1950.

The Reasons for Rising Healthcare Costs

Many reasons have been offered for the disproportionate rise in healthcare costs. Some of the reasons offered are baseless. Others are true, but cannot readily be controlled. A third category consists of causes that are real and controllable. We will focus on the factors that can be controlled, and propose a plan to restore affordability, availability and convenience to American healthcare.

False Explanations for Rising Healthcare Costs

These were addressed in Chapter 2 – Healthcare Myths, so I will only summarize them briefly here:

- *"Technology drives up healthcare costs."* This is simply untrue. Technology naturally drives costs down, except when prevented from doing so by unwise governmental policies and regulations.

- *"Fee-for-service is the problem; we've got to find a better way to pay doctors."* Fee-for-service works fine in every other industry. There is no fundamental reason why it shouldn't work in healthcare too, if incentives weren't distorted by unwise legislation and regulation.

- *"Free markets don't work in healthcare."* As detailed in Chapters 2 and 3, this is a baseless statement. The last time we had anything resembling a free market in healthcare, it consumed 4.5% of GDP, not the nearly 18% it consumes today.

- *"Healthcare warrants extraordinary expenditures because human health and lives are at stake."* The same could be said of food and housing. In truth, public health and lifestyle measures provide more bang for our bucks. The benefit of many (if not most) healthcare expenditures (e.g., doctor visits for the common cold) is marginal at best.

Uncontrollable Reasons for Rising Healthcare Costs

These factors increase healthcare costs, relative to other expense categories, but aren't easily influenced by healthcare policies or legislation.

- *"Unlike manufacturing, software development, and call center work, healthcare labor can't be outsourced.*" This is true. However, it is also true for other sectors in which relative costs have not risen, such as construction, auto and appliance repair, personal services (hair-cutting, house-cleaning, pet-sitting, etc.), and the non-medical professions. This factor plays a minor role.

- A related argument is that "*healthcare labor is not as easily automated as manufacturing.*" This is also true for the previously mentioned industries (construction, etc.) that have not experienced super-inflation. We would likely see more automation and remote management of healthcare services if healthcare over-regulation weren't discouraging innovation and investment.

- "*The increase in the elderly population and the increasing obesity of Americans are driving up healthcare costs.*" These are significant factors. The elderly require much more health services on average, and our senior population is growing. Obesity increases the risk of hypertension, heart disease, stroke, diabetes, degenerative arthritis, cancer, and other diseases. We have been successful in dramatically reducing the rate of smoking, and it is likely that improvements in education and public health measures can control our obesity epidemic. I regard obesity as "uncontrollable" here only with regard to healthcare policy, per se.

Preventable Reasons for Rising Healthcare Costs

We finally arrive at the heart of the matter: what are the real drivers of healthcare inflation that we can control and correct? Here they are, listed approximately in order of decreasing importance.

- ***There is no price competition in healthcare.*** Medicare/Medicaid price-fixing, aped by private insurance, has killed price competition in healthcare. Yes, it's true that insurers "negotiate" fee schedules with "provider networks." But that's like supermarket chains negotiating with food wholesalers, while the prices on supermarket shelves are set by bureaucrats in Washington. Real price competition occurs only when consumers compare prices and vote with their wallets. *Only then can we have efficient matching of goods and services to consumer needs and preferences.*

- ***The consumers of healthcare services are not the payers (the "consumer-payer disconnect").*** Providers are most obligated to please whoever is paying their bills. When consumers are not the payers, they cannot express their preferences and priorities, making it impossible for providers to accommodate them.

- ***Pervasive and overbearing bureaucratic intervention in healthcare doubles the cost of doing business.*** I described in the allegory of Chapter 1 how Medicare's requirements for CPT/ICD coding, compliant documentation, pre-authorization, etc., multiply costs throughout the system.

- ***High barriers to entry for doctors and other providers, hospitals, and new drugs and devices discourage innovation and investment, and prevent competition throughout our healthcare system.***

- ***America's arcane tort system drives up costs.*** Litigation and the fear of litigation encourage over-spending on tests and treatments.

- ***Barriers to self-care increase costs.*** Our current system discourages self-reliance and education in healthcare, and violates our fundamental rights to control and manage our healthcare and our healthcare dollars.

- ***We lack effective electronic medical records (EMRs) and other types of information technology and automation in healthcare.*** Medicare's and other insurers' emphasis on documentation to justify reimbursement has caused EMR vendors to focus on maximizing reimbursement, rather than improving care quality and efficiency.

The good news is that all the items listed above result directly from unwise laws and regulations. Congress can't change the laws of economics, but it can change its own laws, and we The People can change Congress. We *can have abundant, affordable and convenient healthcare in America.* We just have to abolish the laws and regulations that created the current crisis; and replace them with regulations that encourage innovation, competition, efficiency and prosperity.

In virtually every other area of our economy, innovation and free markets have created abundance and affordability. Meanwhile, healthcare has been transformed into a centrally planned economy where prices are fixed, consumers are not allowed to comparison-shop, and suppliers are not allowed to compete on price, reputation and quality. Doctors and hospitals are forced to devote the majority of resources, not to patient care and satisfaction, but to extraneous issues such as "coding," "pre-authorization," and "compliant documentation." Artificial barriers to entry and over-regulation discourage innovation and investment. Price-fixing, insurance abuse and the consumer-payer disconnect prevent competition and discourage economizing at every turn. *There are no mysteries here.*

We simply cannot have abundant and affordable healthcare until we unchain our healthcare system. The system I describe here will in no way diminish Medicare or Medicaid, or decrease healthcare for the poor. On the contrary, because healthcare will be more efficient and affordable, far fewer people will need financial help to obtain it, and taxpayer costs to provide a safety net for the poor will be decreased.

Breaking the Chains

Here are the steps to unchain our healthcare system, and make quality, affordable care available to all. I will start with the basic measures required to restore competition, efficiency and innovation to our healthcare economy. These measures will obviously discombobulate the current medical insurance system and safety net. Bear with me, and those issues will also be resolved. *We can have abundant healthcare for all, and a healthcare system that is the envy of the world.* Here's how.

Breaking the Chains, Part I: Creating an Efficient Healthcare Marketplace

Five steps are essential to create an efficient healthcare marketplace.

1. Free patients to select medical services and products based on quality, reputation and price.

This requires:

- Ending price-fixing, by abolishing Medicare and insurance fee schedules.

- Ending "network contracting." Regardless of insurance, you should be able to choose your doctors, hospitals and other products and services.

- Allowing patients to manage their own healthcare dollars and select whatever doctors and treatments they want, based on costs and benefits relative to their own preferences.

An efficient marketplace responsive to patient needs requires three things:

a) **Transparent Pricing.** State and federal laws should mandate that all licensed providers of medical goods and services post their prices publicly at their places of business, and on the Internet. This simple measure eliminates all cost-shifting.

b) **Reliable Quality Evaluations**. Optimal purchasing requires evaluation of price relative to perceived quality or reputation. In the past, for most goods and services, quality and reputation were evaluated primarily based on individual experience, word-of-mouth and published reviews. Those mechanisms will continue to be important in healthcare.

For our mobile population and growing cornucopia of products and services, the Internet has emerged as a primary source of consumer reviews. Unfortunately, any evaluation system is subject to gaming, and it is estimated that one-third of Internet evaluations are bogus — negative reviews posted by competitors or rave reviews posted by suppliers.

To minimize gaming for Internet evaluations, a federal agency should be created to validate and aggregate healthcare quality ratings and post them on the Internet in a timely manner. There should be stiff penalties for fraudulent evaluations. Options for systematically collecting patient quality reviews include:

   a. Insurance companies could be incentivized or mandated to solicit patient evaluations of the doctors, hospitals and treatments used.
   b. Licensed providers of healthcare goods and services could be incentivized or mandated to solicit patient reviews of all goods and services provided.

Using modern information technology, this could be accomplished with minimal expense.

For example, when a patient checks out after a doctor visit, their discharge instructions would include a unique alphanumeric "key" (e.g., P594-36BQ-U7G9) that the patient could then enter on the official healthcare evaluations website. For a limited time, the key would authorize the patient to fill out an evaluation on that specific doctor. The possibilities are infinite, and a detailed discussion is beyond my objective here.

c) **Economy-Minded Shoppers.** Regardless of their insurance status, patients should be incentivized to comparison-shop. Only then will suppliers be incentivized to offer maximum quality at minimum prices. For out-of-pocket expenses, transparent pricing and quality evaluations are all that is required. Other changes are required for insured and "safety net" purchases. Those changes will be discussed later.

2. Free doctors, clinics and hospitals to compete based on quality, reputation and price.

This requires exactly the same measures listed above to free patients, plus:

- Ridding the world of "CPT coding," "ICD coding," "compliant documentation" and "pre-authorization" requirements. With patients deciding what to buy and how much to pay, these efficiency-killing bad ideas become irrelevant.

Some might object that such coding and documentation have valid medical purposes like quality monitoring and epidemiologic studies. That is arguably true in theory, but in our current system these codes and documentation are worthless for such purposes because:

a) Hurried doctors (or their assistants or billing agents) rarely have time to consider the nuances of specific code definitions. Consequently, they tend to grab any code "in the right ballpark" that they think might get paid.

b) Since reimbursement is based on the codes and documentation, they are heavily "gamed" to maximize reimbursement. Only when documentation has been unchained from reimbursement issues, can it become a useful tool for improving quality and continuity of care, and for supporting research and epidemiologic studies.

These coding and documentation requirements have never contributed anything to our healthcare system but monstrous inefficiency and frustration. Their non-necessity should be clear from a cursory examination of documentation and communications in more efficient sectors. For example, most people have auto and home insurance, and documentation is required for insured expenses. However, you will not find those contracts and documents burdened with thousands of humanly incomprehensible codes and complex documentation rules.

3. Minimize barriers to entry.

An efficient market requires low barriers to entry. For our healthcare market to be efficient, we must make it easier for aspiring young people to become doctors, easier for entrepreneurs to build hospitals and clinics, and easier for inventors to bring new drugs and devices to market. The following measures are needed:

a) The supply of doctors has always been so tightly regulated that only a fraction of qualified applicants have been admitted to medical school. That must end. More medical schools should be built, and enrollment increased at existing schools, until all qualified applicants are able to become physicians. Anyone who wants to and is qualified can become an auto mechanic or a lawyer. The same freedom should apply to physician aspirants.

b) Federal and state laws regarding immigration and licensing of FMGs (foreign medical school graduates) should be liberalized to make it easy for qualified foreign doctors to move to the U.S. and practice here.

c) Laws regulating nurse practitioners, physician assistants and physical therapists should be liberalized, to give them the broadest scope of practice consistent with their education and skills. Schools and enrollment slots for these non-physician practitioners should also be increased to accommodate the increased demand.

d) Laws limiting hospital and clinic construction or expansion, or otherwise limiting innovation and competition, should be repealed.

e) To encourage investment and innovation, the requirement for proof of efficacy for new drugs and devices should be rescinded. Regulation should be limited to the minimum consistent with patient safety. Manufacturers should not be allowed to advertise a new drug or device as both *safe and effective*, until efficacy has been proven. To accomplish that, the FDA should be mandated to evaluate and publish *comparative* efficacy studies; and to specify what efficacy claims manufacturers are allowed to make.

f) We should continue to allow licensed pharmacies in foreign countries to compete on price and quality with U.S. pharmacies. Thus far, current and previous administrations have delayed enforcement of Section 708 of the FDA Safety and Innovation Act, which gives government agencies the authority to seize and destroy safe, imported medications valued at $2500 or less. That section should be repealed.

4. Free patients (and doctors) to care for themselves and their families.

Americans once had the right to treat themselves to whatever extent they were able. We should reclaim that right. In particular:

a) Adult patients who wish to manage their own care should be able to obtain whatever medications they want or need without a prescription.

b) Pharmacists should be encouraged to devote more time and resources to patient education and counseling, and freed from the excessive regulations, pre-authorization and documentation requirements that currently distract them from their proper role. That would largely be accomplished by the price transparency and insurance changes discussed elsewhere in this chapter.

Although prescription laws are highly beneficial to the medical profession's cash flow, they are detrimental to America for multiple reasons:

a) They increase net costs by requiring patients to visit a physician, even when they know perfectly well what they need, or just need refills of a medication they're already using with good results.

b) They encourage dependence on physicians and discourage patients' self-education and self-reliance.

c) They violate our fundamental right to decide for ourselves what to do with our bodies and how to take care of ourselves.

Interestingly, there has been a recent trend toward states limiting *even physicians' right to prescribe for themselves and their families* — not just narcotics, but all prescription medications. Would you prohibit a pilot from flying his own plane, an accountant from doing her own taxes, or a cobbler from shoeing for his own children?

Certainly there are many cases where a physician shouldn't and wouldn't attempt to care for herself or a family member. But these are issues that individuals should be free to address themselves on a case-by-case basis. Blanket prohibitions are symptomatic of an attitude that individuals are incapable of deciding for themselves, and that government knows best. These are not the principals on which this country was founded, and on which it has prospered.

5. Encourage *effective* use of information technology.

Information technology (IT), including EMRs (Electronic Medical Records) can and will increase healthcare quality and efficiency, but *only when and if it evolves naturally in response to business needs*. However, the government can play a critical enabling role in healthcare IT technology, just as it has, for example, in telecommunications.

The proper role of government is not to specify product features, but to ensure a level playing field where all players can freely exchange information. Accordingly, the federal government should sponsor a technology task force comprised of healthcare IT industry leaders, with the following mission, to be accomplished by a reasonable deadline (e.g., in three years):

a) Specify standard data interchange formats, to ensure that all patient health information can be reliably and securely transmitted among all pharmacies, doctors, clinics, and hospitals. This will ensure that any EMR system can exchange data with any other EMR system.

b) Specify a standard, secure and reliable method for making all patient health data immediately accessible on the Internet. This will ensure, for example, that any doctor caring for a patient can instantly access all that patient's past records, no matter where or by whom they were produced.

Breaking the Chains, Part II
Insurance Reform

You don't file an auto insurance claim to fill your gas tank, or use homeowner's insurance to replace a ceiling fan. Why then go to your health insurance company for a flu shot or Pap smear? That simple example shows what a ridiculous creature American health insurance has become. *We cannot have an efficient, affordable healthcare system without restoring insurance to its proper role.* Before discussing reforms, let's briefly recap the major problems with health insurance:

Problems resulting from past abuse of insurance and unwise regulation:

- Insurance use for routine expenses causes a consumer-payer disconnect, removing the patient's incentive to economize. It's also a very inefficient way to finance routine expenditures. Insurance use for routine expenses has been driven by federal rules making it a tax-free form of employee compensation.

- Linking insurance to employment reduces employee mobility, incentivizes employers to avoid hiring people with poor health, and prevents insurance portability.

- Mandated community rating (charging everyone the same premiums, regardless of individual factors) prevents accurate risk pricing, and prevents insurance pricing from incentivizing good health habits. It also incentivizes insurance companies to avoid unhealthy patients, and to over-spend on healthy patients (so as to retain them).

You can think of health insurance as "private sector socialism." It allows many people to voluntarily contribute a little money, so that a lot of money will be available to the few who experience calamities. Insurance companies earn a profit for pricing the risk and providing the infrastructure. To the individual buying insurance, the insurer is selling risk reduction; for society at large, the insurer is redistributing risk.

Insurers will accomplish the desired risk redistribution, whether for not they are mandated to use "community rating." But mandating community rating *prevents* insurance companies from providing another valuable service for society: accurately pricing risk, and thereby incentivizing risk reduction. When insurers are allowed (as in other areas, such as homeowner's and auto insurance) to price insurance based on risk, that provides a strong incentive to the insured to reduce risk, and secondarily to reduce costs.

Prohibiting individual rating has the noble intent to avoid higher premiums for people who incur higher risk through no fault of their own (e.g. with "pre-existing conditions"). But destroying the economic benefit of insurance risk-pricing is *not* a smart way to enhance fairness. It's another example of how adverse unintended consequences of laws often outweigh the benefits.

- The PPACA contains numerous other insurance mandates that, though superficially appealing to voters, will have a net-negative effect on healthcare efficiency, while introducing multitudinous perverse incentives and unintended consequences. For example, mandating that all insurance pay for contraception only "insures" that the price of contraception will not come down during the lifetime of the mandate.

In summary, our current crisis of health insurance affordability results directly from unwise laws and regulations. We do not have similar problems in other areas where counterproductive regulation has not been imposed (e.g., homeowner's and auto insurance). The most important measure is to remove the laws that impose perverse incentives. We discuss this in more detail below.

Problems resulting from the inherent nature of health insurance:

- Unlike with most other forms of insurance (e.g., auto or homeowner's insurance), the risk associated with a patient increases with age, and to a greater degree than for other types of insurance, in proportion to the magnitude of past claims. As with life insurance and many individual health plans, when not prevented by regulations from pricing risk, the insurance industry spontaneously solves this problem with guaranteed renewability — in essence, by providing insurance against your premiums increasing in the future.

- Medical complexity fosters insurance policy complexity. For a homeowner's insurance policy, the types of threats to the house (lightning, tornadoes, flooding, fire, etc.) and the possible means of repair are quite limited. But for health insurance, the number of possible diseases and accidents is enormous, and new tests and treatments are constantly being developed. This is reflected in the relative length and complexity of health insurance contracts compared to, e.g., homeowner's insurance contracts.

  In truth, however, there is no need for health insurance contracts to reflect the multitudinous contingencies of healthcare delivery; and they did not attempt to do so until widespread abuse of insurance caused costs to spiral out of control. If insurance providers were free to provide real insurance, in response to consumer needs, this problem would disappear. An example is given below.

- Healthcare insurance seems prone to egregious practices (e.g., canceling a policy when a patient develops a serious illness). Most "egregious practices" of insurance companies aren't truly egregious, but result from the fact that the contracts are so long and detailed that patients have little idea what isn't covered until the need arises. Laws may be needed to prohibit certain egregious practices, but with the insurance changes described below, insurance agreements would be much simpler, and easy for patients to understand. Consequently, most "egregious practices" would no longer be an issue.

Ideally, health, life, auto, homeowners, renters, and umbrella insurance policies should be quite similar. Health insurance companies should be free to innovate and compete, and individuals should be able to purchase plans for themselves and their families based on their needs and tolerance for risk. Most of the unique problems of health insurance are attributable to the unwise policies of the past, and can be resolved or greatly ameliorated with the following changes.

1. First of all, the perverse tax incentives that have resulted in the common practice of insurance being used for ordinary expenses should be abolished. Ideally, tax-favoring of health expenses should simply be abolished. If you would prefer to spend $25,000 on a new car instead of a new hip joint, why should you have to pay taxes on the car, but not the hip joint? But if that eminently logical notion seems too radical, then tax-free employer-paid contributions to insurance premiums should only be allowed when coupled with tax-free employer-paid contributions to HSAs (Health Savings Accounts, used to pay uninsured out-of-pocket healthcare expenses; see* next paragraph).

    That would encourage employees buy high-deductible insurance (the only kind that meets the definition of *insurance*), and pay for most routine healthcare expenses out-of-pocket (the only way to incentivize smart shopping for routine expenses). Self-employed and unemployed individuals should have the same tax-favored (or not) ability to purchase health insurance and manage HSA accounts.

[*A Health Savings Account (HSA) is a savings account specifically to save for out-of-pocket medical expenses. It is used in combination with a high-deductible insurance policy. The employer makes an automatic tax-free deposit to the HSA every pay period. Any money in the HSA not spent for medical expenses remains in the account, accumulating interest tax-free. The money can be withdrawn for other purposes only by paying income tax plus a 20% penalty. After retirement, the money can be used for other purposes without penalty. A "Roth HSA" is funded with after-tax money, but accumulates interest tax-free.]

2. Insurers should only contract with their true customers: patients. They should not be allowed to contract with providers to be "in network" and accept specific fee schedules. This ensures patients the maximum ability to select the providers and treatments they prefer; and it ensures doctors and hospitals the maximum ability to compete on a level playing field. (If this seems radical, keep in mind that the practices of price-fixing and network contracting only arose in the first place as a response to the perverse incentives and unintended consequences of bad legislation. If we simply removed the perverse incentives that created them, these insurance industry practices

would eventually go away. Unfortunately, by then America might be bankrupt.)

3. To allow insurers to do what they do best — measure and price risk — all mandates for guaranteed issue and community rating must be abolished. Annual and lifetime limits should be variable, based on patients' tolerance for risk and financial status. Rating based on individual risk factors should be permitted, to incentivize risk reduction and minimize net healthcare costs. America's health insurance industry should not be legislatively transformed into a giant, surreptitious income-transfer scheme, or abused by shortsighted legislators as a golden goose.

4. Most "egregious practices" of insurance companies result from the fact that the contracts are so long and detailed that patients don't know (and certainly can't remember) the limits until they bump against them. To avoid patients being blindsided by 57th-page gotcha's, and to avoid frustrating, time-consuming, expensive, confusing and anti-competitive "pre-authorization" issues, insurance contracts should be limited in length and complexity. Like price-fixing and network contracting, most of this complexity was only created to combat the perverse incentives created by unwise legislation and resulting insurance abuse.

In general, exclusions should be limited to specific categories of services or treatments (e.g., cosmetic surgery, obstetric care), to allow policies to match patient needs and risks, without creating incomprehensible complexity. Otherwise, policies should cover all valid bills of licensed providers, subject to deductibles, co-pays, and economizing options to be described later. Such policies would leave all financial, testing and treatment decisions between patients and doctors, within the net constraints of the policy.

With the preceding regulations, patients would have maximum flexibility to shop and choose products and services based on their financial ability and preferences. Providers would be compelled to compete on price and quality. And insurance companies would be freed to produce innovative products that meet patients' needs, while encouraging them to economize.

Let's consider how the above regulations might play out for a typical family with husband, wife, and two children. Assume they don't plan further children, and don't want to pay extra for cosmetic procedure coverage. Assume also that their combined income is $100,000 per year, and they have decided the maximum they can comfortably pay out-of-pocket (not including insurance premiums) is $5000 per year; and that the absolute maximum they want to risk paying in one year, even with an unexpected severe injury or illness, would be $15,000. Also assume that based on estimated current expenses for the most likely severe injuries and illnesses, they are willing to accept an annual limit of $250,000 and a lifetime limit of $5,000,000.

Given the above constraints, this family's best strategy would be to purchase an insurance policy with a deductible of $5000 that excludes coverage for cosmetic procedures and obstetric care. Combined with their reasonable annual and lifetime limits, that should enable them to obtain affordable insurance that leaves them with the maximum ability to manage their healthcare according to their preferences. What other policy features would empower this family and their insurance company to *collaborate* so as to minimize their costs?

One problem with conventional insurance is that, once patients have paid the deductible, they have little or no incentive to economize. If insurers were free to experiment and innovate, our hypothetical family would probably get the best deal with a policy that pays:

a) Nothing for the first $5000 of expenses (the definition of "high deductible").

b) 50% of all expenses between $5000 and $10,000. That significantly incentivizes economizing even above the deductible, while keeping the family's total out-of-pocket expenses down to $7500 if they have $10,000 total expenses.

c) 25% of all expenses between $10,000 and $15,000. That limits total out-of-pocket to $8750 for $15,000 in total expenses.

d) 12.5% of all expenses between $15,000 and $25,000. That limits total out-of-pocket to $10,000 for $25,000 in total expenses.

e) 2% of all expenses from $25,000 to the annual limit of $250,000. That would limit total out-of-pocket expenses to $14,500 even if their expenses totaled $264,500.

f) The policy would have guaranteed renewability, regardless of future health status, for the original premium plus an adjustment for inflation. This feature protects the family from premium increases due to changes in health status as they get older or develop "pre-existing conditions." This "insurance against increased insurance premiums" would, of course, have to be priced according to risk and factored into their initial premium.

The measures we have discussed so far would protect the family against future rate increases, while protecting them from expenses they cannot afford to pay out-of-pocket. Because of the graduated co-payments, the family is incentivized to economize at all levels of expense. Within the net policy constraints, the family and their doctors can choose whatever tests and treatments they prefer, without worrying about whether or not specific items are "covered," and with no pre-authorizations, denials and appeals to worry about.

Much of our current healthcare inefficiency results from the "consumer-payer disconnect," and the graduated co-payments described above ensure that patients retain some "skin in the game" even for large covered expenses. Are there other "economizing levers" that insurance companies could employ to minimize their costs, *without invading the exam room or increasing net system complexity and costs?* Yes, our hypothetical policy would also likely include the following (or similar) features:

g) For non-emergency tests, procedures or treatments with costs above a mutually agreed threshold (perhaps $1500 for our hypothetical family), the insurance company would have the right to obtain three estimates from licensed providers in the patient's area, and cover only the minimum bid. All the patient has to remember is "$1500" to know when an expense must be cleared with their insurance company to avoid additional out-of-pocket costs. Even if the patient chooses not to pre-clear the purchase, she only risks an additional expense equal to the difference between what she pays and the "best bid" the insurance company obtains. Unlike with pre-negotiated fee schedules, insurance companies are empowered to find the best available bargains on a real-time basis, as prices fluctuate. Providers are incentivized to minimize prices on a real-time basis to capture more business.

h) To encourage the family to economize, even for the largest expenses with the minimum 2% co-pay, their premium cost would be subject to increase 0.25% for every $1000 of expense above $25,000. For example, if the family had total costs of $125,000, their rate would increase by ($125,000 - $25,000)/$1000 * 0.25% = 25%. That ensures the family has a significant incentive to economize at all expense levels, to minimize their future premium costs. Because they've selected a policy that is guaranteed renewable, they have an incentive to stay with their current insurance, and to minimize future premium increases.

i) When the patient bargain-shops and pays less than the average price for an item in the area, the insurance company rebates (as cash or future premium discounts) a fraction of the savings. Such practices would be facilitated by the price transparency previously discussed. Note that this feature would encourage patients to investigate prices at emergency departments in their area in advance, so they know where they can get the most affordable care when an emergency arises.

I don't mean to imply that the above features should all be mandated in law. These are just examples of the kind of patient-pleasing, cost-saving innovations that would spontaneously emerge, if insurance companies weren't compelled to do counterproductive things in reaction to perverse incentives resulting from unwise legislation.

To ensure portability and maximize coverage, all policies should be "owned" by the individual or family, not tied to employment or any specific group, and should be portable between states. As previously mentioned, all policies should be tax-favored (or not) regardless of whether obtained through an employer or in the individual market.

Section Summary: I have described what a typical insurance policy might look like, if insurance companies were allowed to design and sell real insurance, and to innovate to meet consumer needs. Such policies would result naturally (and would already dominate the market), had insurers and patients not been consistently subjected to perverse incentives for the past 60 years. Obviously, the unwise regulations and incentives need to be removed. On the other hand, it would not be wise to replace one straightjacket with another. The required reforms are these:

- To allow insurers to do what they do best — measure and price risk so as to most affordably meet specific patient needs — all mandates for first-dollar coverage or coverage of routine expenses, coverage of specific items, community rating, guaranteed issue, and prohibition of policy limits must be abolished.

- Ideally, tax-favoring of health expenses should simply be abolished. If insurance *is* tax-favored, then tax-free contributions to insurance premiums (whether paid by employers or individuals) should be allowed *only* when coupled with tax-free contributions to HSAs (Health Savings Accounts) for out-of-pocket expenses. This avoids incentivizing the abusive practice of using insurance for routine expenses.

- Insurers should only be allowed to contract with their true customers: patients. They should not be allowed to require providers to be "in network" and accept specific fee schedules, etc.

- Insurance contracts should be limited in length and complexity. In general, exclusions should be limited to specific categories of services or treatments (e.g., cosmetic surgery, obstetric care). Otherwise, policies should cover all valid bills of licensed providers, subject to deductibles, co-pays, and other economizing options.

- To maximize the consumer-payer connection and patient responsibility, regulations should encourage:
    - High-deductible policies
    - Graduated co-payments that require some amount of patient contribution even near policy limits.
    - Guaranteed renewability (insurance against increased insurance premiums)
    - Discounts for risk reduction
    - Competitive bidding for big-ticket items
    - Graduated premium increases when total expenses exceed a threshold, to incentivize cost containment at all levels of expense.
    - Savings sharing for bargain purchases.
- All policies should be "owned" by the individual or family, not tied to employment or any specific group.
- All policies should be tax-favored (or not) regardless of whether obtained through an employer or in the individual market.

Breaking the Chains, Part III
A Safety Net for All Americans

Any sensible strategy that aspires to ensure adequate healthcare for all Americans must include these three components:

1. Ending the counterproductive policies of the past, and implementing new policies that encourage an efficient healthcare market. We have discussed how to do this earlier in this chapter.
2. Regulatory policies that encourage individuals and families to save for routine healthcare expenses, and to purchase insurance for major expenses. We discuss this below.
3. A "safety net" to ensure no one suffers from lack of basic healthcare. Note that items 1 and 2 above will ensure that fewer citizens fall into the safety net; and that taxpayers' costs for the safety net are minimized.

Policies to Promote Healthcare Saving and Insurance

To ensure that most employed individuals and their families are insured, employers should be mandated to automatically "opt in" all uninsured hires into an HSA (Health Savings Account) plus a high-deductible insurance (HDI) policy of the employee's choice. (I'll refer to this as an HSA-HDI package.)

The HSA accounts would be handled by banks or other financial institutions, and the insurance policies by licensed insurance companies, so that they travel with the employee when he or she changes employers. The employer's only role is to perform automatic payroll deductions to fund the HSA and pay the insurance premiums. To avoid infringing personal liberties, individuals should be allowed to opt out, but there should be a sufficiently high opt-out hurdle to ensure all but the most ideologically opposed citizens remain in the program.

Similar inducements should be implemented to encourage the self-employed and unemployed to maintain HSA-HDI enrollment. For example:

- Tax preparers could be incentivized to enroll clients in HSA-HDI packages at tax time. Enrollees could be incentivized with one-time tax rebates for enrollment with a commitment to remain enrolled.

- Banks and mortgage lenders could be incentivized to enroll clients in HSA-HDI packages whenever clients open savings, checking or investment accounts, or purchase a new home. Again, enrollees could be incentivized with one-time tax rebates for enrollment with a commitment to remain enrolled.

- Colleges, universities and technical schools could be incentivized to enroll students in HSA-HDI packages, with student incentives for enrollment with a commitment to remain enrolled.

The preceding measures should help ensure that most people who can afford to do so maintain adequate HSA and insurance resources to meet their healthcare needs.

Restructuring the Safety Net

Restructuring the safety net involves two basic components: Medicare for seniors and Medicaid for the poor.

Restructuring Medicare: It should be obvious by now that Medicare in its current form (an "insurance" program with contracted networks and fee schedules) is incompatible with healthcare efficiency and affordability. Accordingly, Medicare must be transformed as quickly as possible into a system where the government makes monthly payments to fund HSA-HDI packages for seniors.

To be politically palatable, such HSA-HDI packages must initially be approximately equivalent, in average net benefits, to the existing program. Over time, as our healthcare system becomes more efficient, greater benefits can be provided for less cost. With these changes, Medicare patients will have access to all doctors, drugs, tests and treatments that are available, without the multitudinous arbitrary restrictions they currently face.

In the revised Medicare system, seniors would be allowed to augment government contributions to their HSA-HDI packages, to increase their benefits or decrease their risks. Younger people should be allowed to opt out of Medicare payroll withholding altogether, if they replace it with an HSA-HDI-pension package that includes guaranteed health insurance in retirement. That will encourage innovation in the private sector to seek optimal solutions to healthcare and pension financing for retirees.

Ultimately, all Medicare and Social Security payroll withholding should be transitioned to private-sector HSA-HDI-pension plans that are federally guaranteed and regulated. Some will object to changing Medicare and Social Security to private-sector plans, claiming that would be an abrogation of the government's obligation to provide some pre-defined level of benefits in the future. But in truth, history proves incontrovertibly that the federal government is not capable of managing its finances to reliably guarantee defined benefits in the future.

As you are probably aware, the federal government has not saved even a fraction of all that we've paid over past decades for our Medicare and Social Security benefits in retirement. All that money, and much more, has been spent. Our federal government owns nothing but a mountain of debt and a printing press. Allowing it to continue to make such commitments only guarantees eventual federal bankruptcy, and subsequent widespread economic pain for our entire nation. Nothing is gained by making promises that are certain to be broken. Properly regulated private institutions are much more likely to responsibly manage our retirement assets than is Congress or the US Treasury.

Restructuring Medicaid: Medicaid suffers from the same fatal problems as Medicare (provider contracting, fee schedules, etc.). It is also plagued with additional perverse incentives that make its costs unmanageable. For example, parents with the option to insure their children through their workplace are incentivized to enroll in Medicaid instead. And Medicaid's common policy of zero-copays for office visits incentivizes frequent doctor visits, driving up costs.

Meanwhile, Medicaid patients are "second-class customers." The fees are so low that many doctors do not take Medicaid patients, restricting their options. Offices that accept Medicaid patients often give them the lowest priority for appointments and for staff attention, to provide better service for better-paying customers. Also, drug coverage is severely restricted for Medicaid patients, relative to Medicare and private insurance.

The solution for Medicaid is simple, and similar to the solution for Medicare. Individuals and families that fall below an income threshold should be eligible for government subsidized HSA-HDI packages. The subsidies would be sufficient to fund benefits equal or better than average current Medicaid benefits, but would have several advantages. Since all family members, regardless of employment status, would be included in the same HSA-HDI package, problems with parents avoiding contributions through the workplace in order to access Medicaid benefits would be avoided. Families would retain the same HSA-HDI package as their financial status changes, weaning off subsidies and beefing up their benefits as their employment or financial status improves.

This approach to Medicaid would allow government agencies to flexibly adjust benefits, depending on economic conditions and availability of funds. Patients would pay for services with EBT (electronic benefits transfer) cards that are valid only for healthcare products and services, similar to the EBT cards used by SNAP ("food stamp") beneficiaries.

Medicaid patients would have the same incentives to economize as self-funded patients. Limits on their HSA funds and insurance benefits would encourage smart shopping. As with patient-financed HSA-HDI packages, unspent funds in their HSAs would accumulate for future healthcare needs or retirement. Their insurance policies would have the same incentives as self-paid policies.

Medicaid patients would be eligible to use the same doctors, services and drugs as anyone else, but their net benefits would typically be less than with self-funded HSA-HDI packages. That would maximize their incentives to economize, while encouraging providers to offer lower-cost, no-frills services and products, to access that market segment.

Some will object that I am describing a two-tiered system: one for the poor, and another for everyone else. We should not let our ideology obscure reality. We *already have* a two-tiered system where Medicaid patients get the scraps. The system I have described will result in the greatest healthcare abundance, *including for those who must rely on government largesse*. To continue down our current path is certain to result in a two-tiered system where everyone who can afford it uses "concierge medicine," and everyone else is doomed to deteriorating service in our deteriorating system.

Ancillary Measures to
Reduce Healthcare Costs

The measures discussed above would make healthcare in America efficient, affordable, available and convenient. Those measures would also do much to restore solvency to federal and state governments. Several other measures are also important, and would probably achieve at least another 20% net reduction in healthcare costs.

1. Tort Reform

It is estimated that tort reform could reduce healthcare costs by 5-10%, though estimates vary widely. In our current climate, most doctors practice "defensive medicine" to one degree or another, because nearly every doctor has been sued, or has a close friend or colleague who's been sued.

It's hard to imagine the psychological impact of a malpractice suit. Even if the doctor knows he is blameless, the Sheriff still confronts him publicly in his hospital, in front of nurses, janitors, colleagues and patients, to serve the subpoena. Even if blameless, the doctor still gets grilled by the plaintiff's attorneys — digging, probing, insinuating, to find or implicate every possible flaw in his knowledge, logic or character. Even when blameless, the doctor still wonders… will his reputation be ruined? Will he be financially ruined? Will patients and colleagues desert him?

I will describe a real malpractice suit to which I was privy, because it illustrates the major flaw in our current tort system. Only the names are fictional. Briefly, a 60-year-old gentleman having a myocardial infarction (an "MI" or "heart attack") was brought to the ER at St. Mary's Hospital by ambulance. The ER doctor, Dr. Smith, diagnosed and treated him properly, but nonetheless he experienced a "cardiac arrest" not long after arrival. The arteries to his heart were so severely blocked by a clot that his heart could no longer function. Despite the best efforts of Dr. Smith and the St. Mary's ER team, the patient could not be resuscitated, and he died in the ER. If that were the extent of his medical care that day, his family would not have sued anyone. But he didn't go to St. Mary's first.

Instead, he had gone to a different hospital (we'll call it St. Anne's) several hours previously. The doctor at that hospital, despite obvious signs of myocardial infarction on his EKG, diagnosed "peptic ulcer disease" and sent him home with a prescription for ulcer medicine. Several hours later, when his pain got worse, he called 911 and had the paramedics take him to St. Mary's. But by then, the window of opportunity to save his life was already closing. Had the first doctor diagnosed his MI and administered the routine "clot-busting drugs" earlier that day, his heart and his life would probably have been saved.

The doctor who sent the patient home with a prescription for ulcer medication was clearly guilty of malpractice. However, this patient's family (the "plaintiffs") didn't sue just the guilty doctor. They sued:

1. the doctor at St. Anne's who misdiagnosed him and sent him home,
2. St. Anne's Hospital, where he was first seen,
3. Dr. Smith, the ER doctor at St. Mary's, where he died shortly after admission to the ER,
4. St. Mary's Hospital, and
5. the ambulance service that transported him.

Why did they sue not only the culpable physician, but also four other entities? For one reason only: in our current system, the more people you sue, the more money you're likely to get; and *there is no downside to suing everyone in sight.*

So what happened? Dr. Smith was served by the Sheriff at his hospital, in front of nurses, janitors, colleagues and patients. He was grilled by the plaintiff's attorneys at deposition — digging, probing, insinuating, to expose every possible flaw in his knowledge, logic and character. But he never got his day in court. He was never "exonerated." He never got an apology, much less thanks for his efforts to save the patient's life.

After six years of closed-door negotiations among the opposing attorneys, the case was settled out-of-court for a total payment of approximately $100,000. Most of the payment was made on behalf of the ER doctor at St. Anne's, who misdiagnosed the heart attack. Lesser amounts were paid by the two hospitals and the ambulance service. No contribution was made on behalf of Dr. Smith.

Why was Dr. Smith accused when there was no evidence of malpractice on his part? For two simple reasons:

1. Doctors (or their insurance companies) will often pay a substantial amount, just to dispel the ominous cloud hanging over their head, or to avoid the risk of a much larger judgment if the case goes to court. Even if a doctor is blameless, it takes years for a case to go to court. And no matter how blameless the defendant, the plaintiff's attorneys can always

find an incompetent doctor who no longer practices medicine, and is happy to testify against a colleague for a handsome fee. Regardless of the doctor's culpability, juries are often swayed by the emotional trauma of the family who has lost a loved one. *Even if a doctor is blameless, going to court is a long tribulation and a big risk.*

2. Plaintiffs and their attorneys risk nothing by suing a blameless doctor. Even though blameless, Dr. Smith never got his day in court. The plaintiffs didn't have to pay his attorney's fees and litigation costs. They didn't have to pay for his wasted time and lost sleep.

The solution to this problem is simple: *All states should enact the "loser pays rule" for medical malpractice cases* (and for torts suits in general, for that matter). If the plaintiffs had known they would have to pay Dr. Smith's expenses if they lost, it is highly unlikely they would have sued him, because they knew they had a weak case. They would still have sued the guilty doctor, because they had a strong case against him. But they would not have dragged Dr. Smith into it, just on the off-chance they might extort another few thousand bucks, risk free.

If plaintiff patients and their attorneys knew they would have to pay out when their bluff fails, they'd be far less inclined to bet; doctors would sleep much better; and our total healthcare costs would probably decline another 5-10%.

2. Stop poisoning the poor with free food!

When the "food stamps" program was created in 1939, the intent was to re-direct farm surplus to under-nourished city dwellers. Today we still have malnutrition, but not due to lack of food. Today's problem is the opposite: too much food. As the obesity epidemic spreads from the US worldwide, so do obesity related illnesses, including hypertension, cardiovascular disease, diabetes, stroke and cancer. The obesity problem is particularly severe in low-income families. Obesity is now the only significant childhood nutritional problem in America, and even type II diabetes, previously rare in children, is on the rise.

The current federal food stamp program, SNAP (Supplemental Nutrition Assistance Program) does not have any nutritional standards. In 2010 federal officials rejected a proposal by New York City to exclude sweetened beverages from the program in spite of the fact that SNAP recipients typically consume 40% more sweetened beverages than any other consumer group. Statistics show that every year of participation in SNAP increases the BMI (Body Mass Index, a measure of obesity) by 1.6 points. Other studies point to the positive association between excess weight and food assistance [40].

Today, if there is any single simple measure that would reliably improve the health of the poor (and every other economic class, for that matter), it would be to *eat less food*! So why is our government giving away *75 billion dollars of free food every year*? [24] It *might* make sense to give out vouchers for *fresh and fresh-frozen produce*, but giving obese people carte-blanche at America's supermarkets is not helping the poor. It is only adding to their health problems, and increasing our healthcare costs.

3. End the "War on Drugs"

It would be reasonable to outlaw addictive drugs, if making them illegal decreased drug use and addiction. But it doesn't. It only creates multiple additional problems that, collectively, cost America *at least 100 billion dollars* annually, and probably two or three times that much if you consider the hidden costs.

1. Roughly half of the people in federal prison are there for drug-related offenses. Not only is the cost of incarcerating them enormous, but their families usually become dependent on government aid during their incarceration. Once released from prison, a criminal record makes it difficult to find employment, and greatly decreases their chance of becoming working, law-abiding citizens.

2. Our current epidemics of AIDS and chronic hepatitis C (both very expensive chronic diseases) are caused primarily by the fact that drug addicts are forced to satisfy their cravings surreptitiously.

3. We are not winning the war on drugs. All we are doing is creating a thriving underground economy in America that makes a life of crime appear the quickest and most glamorous path to prosperity for a million directionless young people.

4. Primary care physicians squander a significant fraction of their professional time and

organizational resources dealing with "drug seekers" attempting to obtain narcotics under false pretenses. From my experience as a primary care doctor, I estimate that roughly 10% of patient encounters involve patients feigning or exaggerating symptoms to obtain narcotic prescriptions. For patients with insurance, Medicare or Medicaid, such encounters often result in thousands of dollars spent trying to diagnose non-existent medical problems.

It is a national embarrassment that our "American Addiction" is fueling narcotics trafficking, terrorism and gangsterism around the world, and is responsible for the murders of thousands of innocent Central and South Americans caught in the crossfire. History has proven repeatedly that banning addictive substances is futile. So why does our government persist in this fabulously expensive and internationally embarrassing folly? The implications are obvious:

a) All addictive substances should be decriminalized.

b) All addictive substances with significant health or safety impacts should be controlled similar to alcohol and tobacco (e.g., to prevent sale to minors and to ensure proper labeling and product consistency).

c) All addictive substances with significant health or safety impacts should be taxed at a rate sufficient to pay for the damage done, but not high enough to create a black market.

Isn't it time we treated all addictive drugs similar to the way we treat the *two most addictive and health-damaging drugs of all* — alcohol and tobacco?

Chapter Summary

The most essential measures to restore efficiency, affordability, availability and innovation to our healthcare system are these:

1. Free patients to select doctors and hospitals based on quality, reputation and price.
2. Free doctors, clinics and hospitals to compete based on quality, reputation and price.
3. Minimize barriers to entry for doctors, hospitals, insurance companies, pharmaceutical companies and device makers.
4. Free patients (and doctors) to care for themselves and their families.
5. Encourage effective use of information technology.
6. Change the perverse tax incentives that have contributed to the current crisis.
7. Restore the true definition of insurance, uncouple insurance from employment, and free insurance companies to meet patient needs and preferences.
8. Revise Medicare and Medicaid in accordance with the same principles.

Ancillary measures that I estimate would decrease health care costs at least an additional 20% include:

1. Enact real tort reform.

2. Stop poisoning the poor with free food.
3. End the "War on Drugs."

Conclusion

Healthcare costs have been rising much faster than inflation for decades, as a direct result of unwise legislation. At every step, as the damage became apparent, instead of correcting past mistakes Congress has layered on more unwise legislation. The latest "reforms," embodied in the 2011 Patient Protection and Affordable Care Act, only continue that trend.

Contrary to American ideals of freedom and liberty, the PPACA goes farther than Medicare and Medicaid to limit the options and infringe the freedoms of patients, doctors and businesses. Moreover, contrary to America's proven economic success with free markets in other economic domains, the PPACA mandates central bureaucratic management and price-fixing policies that can only lead to further economic stagnation and national poverty.

Consequently, we have arrived at a state where:

1. Nobody — not doctors, patients, insurers, pharmaceutical companies or technology suppliers — knows the true value of healthcare goods and services. Furthermore, no one much cares, *as long as someone else is paying*.

2. More time and resources are spent determining what can be paid for, and by whom, and according to what rules, than is actually spent providing care.

3. Healthcare now costs at least twice what it could and would cost in a competitive economy.

4. Healthcare has now become so inefficient and expensive that it is literally bankrupting our nation.

We cannot have affordable healthcare and a prosperous economy, unburdened by exorbitant healthcare costs, until:

1. *Doctors, hospitals, medical suppliers and insurance companies compete based on quality and price.*
2. *Patients take responsibility for managing their health and their healthcare expenses.*
3. *The real definition of "insurance" is restored: protection against catastrophic events.*

To believe otherwise is to ignore the lessons of recent history and economics, and continue down our current path toward national bankruptcy.

We *can* achieve healthcare abundance and put America back on the path to prosperity and international preeminence. I have outlined the necessary steps above. They are not numerous or complex. But implementing them will be difficult because many special interests and industries have become addicted to, or invested in, the waste and inefficiency of the current system.

Fixing our healthcare system and restoring our prosperity will not be easy. Neither was inventing the airplane, winning World War II, walking on the moon, or developing the Internet. We have a history of solving big problems.

As Winston Churchill said, "You can always count on Americans to do the right thing — after they've tried everything else." We've tried everything else. It's time to do the right thing. Let us begin.

References

[1] HSC Community Tracking Study Physician Survey in 1996-97, 1998-99 and 2000-01. Center for Studying Health System Change.

[2] Losing Ground: Physician Income, 1995–2003. Center for Studying Health System Change.

[3] Relationship Between Regional Per Capita Medicare Expenditures and Patient Perceptions of Quality of Care. Floyd J. Fowler Jr, PhD, et al. JAMA. 2008; 299(20):2406-2412.

[4] National Health Spending in 2005: The Slowdown Continues. Aaron Catlin, et al, and the National Expenditure Health Accounts Team, Health Affairs, January/February 2007, Vol. 26, No. 1, pp.142-153.

[5] Medical Expenditures during the Last Year of Life: Findings from the 1992-1996 Medicare Current Beneficiary Survey. Hoover, Donald R., et al. Health Services Research. 37: December, 2002:1625-1642.

[6] Wikipedia definition of "insurance." http://en.wikipedia.org/wiki/Insurance

[7] 'The Cause of My Life' - Inside the fight for universal health care. By Edward M. Kennedy. Newsweek, Issue date July 27, 2009.

[8] Lifestyle Risk Factors and New-Onset Diabetes Mellitus in Older Adults. The Cardiovascular Health Study. Dariush Mozaffarian, et al. Arch Intern Med. 2009; 169(8): 798 807.

[9] Lifestyle Risk Factors Predict Healthcare Costs in an Aging Cohort. J. Leigh, H. Hubert, P. Romano.

American Journal of Preventive Medicine, Volume 29, Issue 5, Pages 379-387.

[10] 111TH CONGRESS; 1ST SESSION H. R. 3200; (A Bill) To provide affordable, quality health care for all Americans and reduce the growth in health care spending, and for other purposes. Full text available at
http://energycommerce.house.gov/Press_111/20090714/aahca.pdf
and also at
http://www.opencongress.org/bill/111-h3200/text

[11] Flatlined - Resuscitating American Medicine. Guy L Clifton, M.D. Rutgers University Press, 2009.

[12] H. R. 3962 To provide affordable, quality health care for all Americans and reduce the growth in health care spending, and for other purposes.
http://docs.house.gov/rules/health/111_ahcaa.pdf

[13] Bending the Cost Curve. http://cboblog.cbo.gov

[14] Memo to the Supreme Court: Health Care Is Not a Right. Richard M. Salsman, Forbes, 4/03/2012.
http://www.forbes.com/sites/richardsalsman/2012/04/03/memo-to-the-supreme-court-health-care-is-not-a-right/

[15] More Doctors Giving Up Private Practices. Gardiner Harris, The New York Times, March 25, 2010.
http://www.nytimes.com/2010/03/26/health/policy/26docs.html?pagewanted=1&fta=y

[16] An Experimental Study of Competitive Market Behavior. Vernon Smith, Journal of Political Economy 30, no. 2 (1962): 111–137.

[17] The Prevalence and Effects of Occupational Licensing. Morris Kleiner and Alan Krueger, British Journal of Industrial Relations 48, no. 4 (2010): 676–687.

[18] Certificate of Need: State Health Laws and Programs. National Conference of State Legislatures, http://www.ncsl.org/issues-research/health/con-certificate-of-need-state-laws.aspx (accessed May 2012).

[19] Saving Capitalism From the Capitalists: Unleashing the Power of Financial Markets to Create Wealth and Spread Opportunity. Raghuram Rajan and Luigi Zingales, New York: Crown Business, 2003.

[20] The Theory of Economic Regulation. George Stigler, Bell Journal of Economics and Management Science 2, (1971): 3–21.

[21] The Pathology of Privilege: The Economic Consequences of Government Favoritism. Matthew Mitchell, Jul 08, 2012. http://mercatus.org/publication/pathology-privilege-economic-consequences-government-favoritism

[22] Private Insurance Is More Efficient than Medicare–By Far. Michael F. Cannon. http://www.cato-at-liberty.org/private-insurance-is-more-efficient-than-medicare-by-far/

[23] Is Medicare More Efficient Than Private Insurance? John Goodman and Thomas Saving. http://healthaffairs.org/blog/2011/08/09/is-medicare-more-efficient-than-private-insurance/

[24] Supplemental Nutrition Assistance Program Participation and Costs (Data as of August 30, 2012).

United States Department of Agriculture Web site.
http://www.fns.usda.gov/pd/SNAPsummary.htm

[25] The Righteous Mind. Jonathan Haidt, 2012. Pantheon Books. For an incisive brief excerpt, see "Why you vote the way you do" in The Week, MAY 25, 2012:
http://theweek.com/article/index/228375/why-you-vote-the-way-you-do

[26] Who Really Cares: The Surprising Truth About Compassionate Conservatism. Arthur C. Brooks and Dennis Holland.

[27] Flexner Report, Wikipedia.
http://en.wikipedia.org/wiki/Flexner_Report

[28] Harrison Narcotics Tax Act, Wikipedia.
http://en.wikipedia.org/wiki/Harrison_Narcotics_Tax_Act

[29] A History of the FDA and Drug Regulation in the United States (a timeline history on the FDA website).
http://www.fda.gov/downloads/Drugs/ResourcesForYou/Consumers/BuyingUsingMedicineSafely/UnderstandingOver-the-CounterMedicines/ucm093550.pdf

[30] History of the FDA (on the official FDA website).
http://www.fda.gov/AboutFDA/WhatWeDo/History/default.htm

[31] History of Federal Regulation: 1902–Present. The Independent Institute. (A Libertarian view of FDA history.) http://www.fdareview.org/history.shtml

[32] The Complexities of Physician Supply and Demand: Projections Through 2025. Michael J. Dill and Edward S. Salsberg, Center for Workforce Studies, Association of American Medical Colleges, November

2008.
http://www.innovationlabs.com/pa_future/1/background_docs/AAMC%20Complexities%20of%20physician%20demand,%202008.pdf

[33] Malpractice Lawsuits in the US: Trends over Time and How Recent Reductions in Damage Awards Could Change Medicine. Yale Journal of Medicine and Law, Vol. VIII, Issue 1.
http://www.yalemedlaw.com/2011/12/malpractice-lawsuits-in-the-us-trends-over-time-and-how-recent-reductions-in-damage-awards-could-change-medicine/

[34] Medical Malpractice: The Good, the Bad, and the Ugly. Kevin R. Loughlin, MD, MBA. Urol Clin N Am 36 (2009) 101–110.
http://inovapeds.org/library/readings/Liability/Medical%20Malpractice%20-%20The%20Good,%20the%20Bad,%20and%20the%20Ugly.pdf

[35] The Unanticipated Consequences of Purposive Social Action. Merton, Robert K, 1936. American Sociological Review 1 (6): 894–904.

[36] An Inquiry into the Nature and Causes of the Wealth of Nations. Adam Smith, 1776.

[37] Basic Economics – A Common Sense Guide to the Economy (4th Edition). Thomas Sowell, 2011.

[38] Priceless: Curing the Healthcare Crisis (Independent Studies in Political Economy). John C. Goodman, 2012.

[39] The Legislative History of the Durham-Humphrey Amendments and the Consideration of Social Harms in the Rx-OTC Switch. Gregory W. Reilly, 2006. Legal

Electronic Document Archive of Harvard Law School.
http://leda.law.harvard.edu/leda/data/787/Reilly06.html

[40] Obesity Among Poor Americans: Is Public Assistance the Problem? Smith, P., 2009. Vanderbilt University Press.

[41] Blue Cross Blue Shield Association. Wikipedia.
http://en.wikipedia.org/wiki/Blue_Cross_Blue_Shield_Association

[42] Cut Medicine in Half. Robin Hanson, Cato Institute. *Cato Unbound*, September, 10th, 2007.
http://hanson.gmu.edu/cutmed.htm

[43] What Did Medicare Do? The Initial Impact of Medicare on Mortality and Out of Pocket Medical Spending. Amy Finkelstein and Robin McKnight. Journal of Public Economics 92 (2008): 1644-1669.

[44] Free for All?: Lessons from the Rand Health Insurance Experiment. Joseph P. Newhouse. Cambridge: Harvard University Press. 1993.

[45] Covering the Uninsured: How Much Would It Cost? Jack Hadley and John Holahan, *Health Affairs* 22(2003).

[46] Readers Speak Out on Solo Practice. Brandi White. Family Practice Management 1998 May; 5(5):58-74. American Academy of Family Physicians web site: http://www.aafp.org/fpm/1998/0500/p58.html

[47] Institute of Medicine November 9, 2009 Rosenthal Lecture, by the Hon. David M. Walker.

About the Author

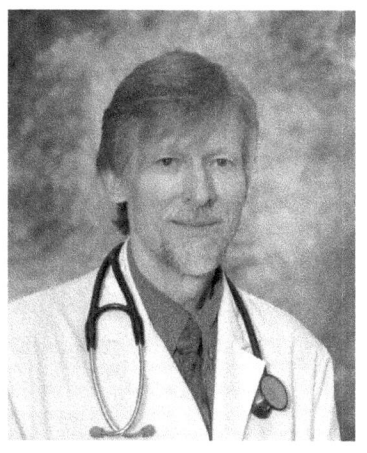

I was born in Memphis, Tennessee in 1953. My dad was a chemical engineer and a Southern Baptist minister. In the late 1950s, he was ousted from his pulpit for inviting the black folks in our community to attend our church. He taught me to do the right thing first, and worry about the consequences later. My mom was a social worker at the Memphis public hospital and Le Bonheur Children's Hospital. I grew up in the rural Arkansas delta and Memphis, Tennessee, with two brothers and one sister.

I graduated from Rhodes College in Memphis with a degree in Chemistry, and got my M.D. at the University of Tennessee College of the Health Sciences in 1980. I am board certified in emergency medicine.

During my first year of medical school, while lost in the medical library late one night, I had an epiphany that has shaped my career. I realized I was swimming in a sea of information that would make me an incredibly good doctor — *if I could learn it all*. Sadly, I realized I could never learn it all. It's just too much for any human to master. At the same time, I was encouraged by the insight that healthcare is not limited by our *knowledge*, but only by the limited capacity of our brains to store and apply that knowledge. I was intrigued by the notion that computing technology — still primitive in 1977 — might allow us to transcend those barriers in my lifetime.

In subsequent years, I practiced emergency medicine and founded Challenger Corporation, with the goal of using information technology to improve physician education. Later, I opened a small-town primary care clinic, where I practiced for 9 years, developed software to improve clinic efficiency, and struggled to survive in a world of disappearing small practices. That experience demonstrated vividly how inefficient our healthcare system has become, and challenged me to seek solutions.

When not working on healthcare technology or policy, I enjoy hiking, yoga, music and reading. My wife, Alicia, and I live in northwest Arkansas. We are currently developing medical software tools to improve healthcare access and delivery. I can be reached at dan.unchained@gmail.com.

Yours for Better Healthcare,

Dan Jones, MD

www.ingramcontent.com/pod-product-compliance
Lightning Source LLC
Chambersburg PA
CBHW061508180526
45171CB00001B/83